D0939943

What The U.S. Healthcare System Doesn't Want ~~You~~ To ~~Know~~

+ Why, And How You Can Do Something About It ←

THOUGHT COLLECTION PUBLISHING
P.O. Box 2132
Naperville, IL. 60540
www.thoughtcollection.org

Copyright © 2019 Kat Lahr

All Rights Reserved. This book or any portion thereof may not be reproduced or used in any matter whatsoever without the express written permission of the publisher except for the use of brief quotations in a book review. For permission requests, contact the publisher at the contact information above.

The To Err Is Healthcare Series, Thought Collection Publishing, and colophon are trademarks of Stellation Group, LLC.

Editing by Miranda Malinowski
Design by Davis Smith at www.DavisSmithDesign.com

First Edition, 2019

Printed in the United States of America

Library of Congress Control Number: 2019912481

Paperback ISBNs:
B & W - 13: 978-1-7334685-2-7
Color - 13: 978-0-9966635-8-8

Hardcover ISBNs:
B & W - 13: 978-1-7334685-3-4
Color - 13: 978-1-7334685-4-1

Digital ISBNs:
EPUB - 13: 978-1-7334685-0-3
MOBI - 13: 978-1-7334685-1-0

We hope you enjoy this book, a part of the To Err Is Healthcare series, meant to create awareness in healthcare consumers.

What The U.S. Healthcare System Doesn't Want You To Know, Why, And How You Can Do Something About It

In An Effort To Inform The American People

Kat Lahr

Thought Collection Publishing

Chicago, Illinois

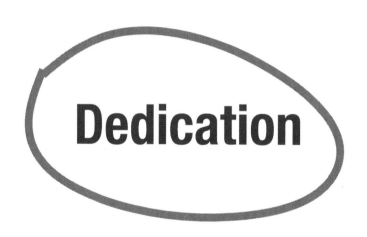

Dedication

To my kids, for showing me the true value of healthcare.

Table of Contents

Foreword

In the absence of the truth, all of us stand helpless to defend ourselves, our families and our health, which is the greatest gift we have. - Erin Brockovich

In 2011, I embarked on a research journey in an attempt to understand the United States healthcare system. I was exhausted from receiving conflicting information about reform efforts, and I wanted to understand it on my own. I was a professor in charge of educating students, so I felt it was my duty to better understand the vast and complex healthcare industry. I started by collecting stories from people of their experiences within the healthcare system. Not only were people willing to tell me their stories, I was shocked at the breadth of them all. Stories ranged from interactions with specialists to billing misunderstandings, awful customer service, process inadequacies, and much more. I often would hear opinions about how awful the Affordable Care Act (ACA), or Obamacare, as it's generally known, is through a misguided lens of a person who didn't fully understand what the law was about. As a professor that taught healthcare law at the time, it was painful to see how many people didn't truly know what was going on in healthcare, a system that we spend our entire lives interacting with. Instead, their opinions were framed by their generally terrible experiences and conditioned thinking about the law and how it affected them. I also received stories from people who were negatively affected by our healthcare system, ones whose voices rang clear to me that we are not done reforming.

Between the unintentional consequences of our healthcare laws and the intentionally misguided public, I was fueled to research more. So I did, and in this book, I am reviewing a small portion of this research and the subsequent conclusions I have made because of it. I have to emphasize that these are my conclusions, and you may come to different ones. That's totally fine. The purpose of this book is to expose you to this data, so you can process it, and make your own conclusions—the first step to becoming an informed health consumer. According to research studies on health literacy by the National Assessment of Adult Literacy, roughly only 10-12% of the general population is aware of the information I'm about to share with you. It is my belief that in order for our healthcare system to change for the better, this number needs to rise. Change is in our hands and within our reach, but it starts with consumer pressure.

My overall objective for this book is to inform and spark conversation about healthcare within the general public. Having the conversation in the first place is an immediate win in our favor. In alignment with a genuine search for truth, this book aims to provide a snapshot of the core dialogue taking place in our healthcare system, especially outside of mainstream channels. Let the data in this book take you where it needs to in your world. I don't expect you to blindly follow the thoughts I express in my bold claims; instead, my aim is to provide a platform for you to launch into your own investigation and discussion around these and other related matters. The reality is that those who benefit from maintaining the status quo are likely to reject any competing ideas. However, through examining data and evidence, we can cautiously weigh the various arguments and perspectives; our duty is in discerning what's more aligned with the truth than what's not.

Part 1

What Does Healthcare Want ~~You~~ (You)

The U.S System Not To ~~Know~~ ?

Before starting, please take five minutes to reflect upon the quote on the following page. Feel free to use the space provided below to write, draw or sketch anything that comes to your mind.

"Radical simply means grasping things at the root."
— Angela Davis

Chapter 1

An Alarming Landscape

Healthcare *is* a complex word.

Partially because it's defined differently by people and organizations depending on income, place of employment, political affiliation, address, age, and much more. But also, it's a fundamentally large part of our lives. We are born into, live, and die in the system without choice. We are born to need healthcare. It's necessary for us to regularly maintain our health, and we often need medical services of some sort to assist us with that. Whether that's having open heart surgery to fix a congenital defect upon birth, using an inhaler to control asthma, or purchasing vitamins to get rid of a deficiency, the healthcare system is embedded heavily in our daily lives. Something so personal to our lives makes a world of difference in how the word is defined. As a person of study, I found that the best way to get a better understanding of the healthcare system in the U.S. is to compare it with other countries.

- -

How do other humans around the world deal with healthcare?

Across the world we all cannot agree on a lot of things because of different beliefs and cultures accustomed to societies, but one thing most nations can agree on is that healthcare is a right. On December 10, 1948, forty-eight countries agreed to the *United Nations' Universal Declaration of Human Rights*.

Article 25 of that document notes the right to healthcare:

> $\rightarrow$ *"Everyone has the right to a standard of living adequate for the health and well-being of himself and of his family, including food, clothing, housing, and medical care and necessary social services."* $\leftarrow$

Today, almost 200 nations have agreed to this statement for a total of 30 articles universally protecting the rights a person has because they are human.

Universal Healthcare *sets* **a standard for which all societies should pursue in order to maintain humanity's fundamental needs.**

↓

"35 of today's 36 developed nations *have* universal health coverage with the U.S. being the *only* exception."

→ ← ↑

Source: Organisation for Economic Co-operation and Development (OECD)

In response to signing this agreement, leaders from developed nations with the finances available have gone back to their respective countries and implemented universal healthcare as a form of social responsibility to this declaration.

According to data monitored by the Organization for Economic Co-operation and Development (OECD), 35 of today's 36 developed nations have universal health coverage with the U.S. being the only exception.

Universal healthcare is the norm for industrialized nations.

Even though Eleanor Roosevelt, the wife of U.S. President Franklin Roosevelt, was Chair of the United Nations Commission that wrote the Universal Declaration of Human Rights in 1948, the U.S. still stands alone within the developed world in efforts to make healthcare available to all of their citizens.

An Alarming Landscape

This means that healthcare is, instead, treated as a commodity, not a right. It's something we have to buy, a privilege, and a benefit. It's not something you get just for being born in the U.S. as you would if born in other countries, such as in Poland, Slovenia, Finland, or France.

Instead, access to healthcare in the U.S. is through insurance, which provides an entire slew of limitations including affordability, subpar plans, risk of bankruptcy, and more.

Since the U.S. takes a different approach with our healthcare system, we stand out in almost every health metric in comparison to the rest of the developed world.

One important metric is how much money countries spend on healthcare—total health expenditure as a percent of Gross Domestic Product (GDP). The OECD 2019 health data shows the U.S. coming in at 17% of our GDP being spent on health expenditures with the next closest countries being Switzerland and France at 12% and 11% and most others between 8-9%.

This means that over 17% of our economy is directed towards healthcare. This equates to a per person health spending of $10,586 in the U.S., which is 60% higher than the average of all OECD countries at $4,000, with our neighbor Canada at $4,974.

As one of the wealthiest countries in the world, the U.S. is expected to spend more money on healthcare, but OECD health data has been adjusted for cost of living differences.

It's our *commodity-based* model that <u>forces</u> us to stand *apart* from the rest.

An Alarming Landscape

This point is even more pronounced when looking at the source of funding for that $10,586 per person health spending. The following study by The Commonwealth Fund shows that we are already paying what other countries pay for Universal Health Coverage—except we don't have it.

Instead, it shows that our current privatized and fragmented commodity-based healthcare system costs more than public healthcare for other countries around the world.

I must repeat this; we are already paying for the cost of Universal Healthcare and then some. ⭐

One big difference is that the U.S. has this huge additional cost called health insurance or private health spending. The per capita spending chart shows that our current private, insurance-based healthcare system costs more than public healthcare.

If you are curious as to how many other countries deal with private health insurance at all, it's not a lot.

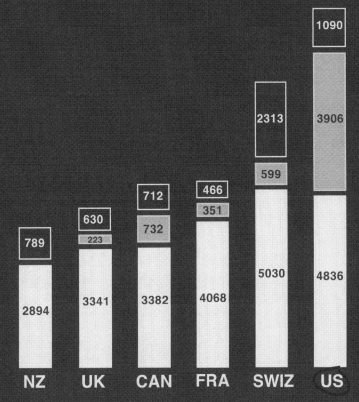

Healthcare Spending Per Capita By Source Of Funding, 2017

In U.S. Dollars & Adjusted for Differences in Costs of Living

Public Spending — Private Spending — Out of Pocket Spending

Source: Organisation for Economic Co-operation and Development (OECD) Health Data. 2018

An Alarming Landscape

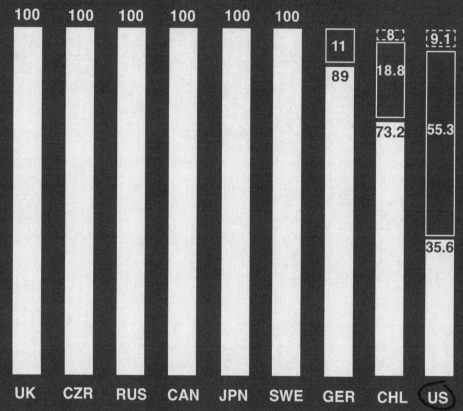

Population Coverage for Core Set of Services, 2017

In Percentage of the Total Population

Uninsured   Private Health Coverage   Total Public Coverage

Source: Organisation for Economic Co-operation and Development (OECD) Health Data. 2015

The private health insurance-based model is very much embedded in the U.S. system and not many others. OECD health data points out that only a total of five of the 37 countries studied deals with private health insurance for primary coverage. The U.S. has the highest rate at 55% with the next closest country being Chile at almost 19%.

The rest of the 32 countries utilize public programs for their primary care coverage.

More people in the U.S. go *without* access to primary healthcare than in *most other developed countries* due to the largely privatized system.

Chapter 2

Counting
Our
Costs

As a *result* of the U.S.

...having the highest usage of private health insurance as our primary coverage, it costs more for us to administer it. Just as retailers are forced to have higher prices on the products they sell because they are making up for distributor and wholesale costs, private health insurance adds an additional layer of cost in a similar fashion.

Instead of doing it ourselves, we pay an insurance company to manage our health benefits, pay our claims, and more. Administrative costs needed to run healthcare businesses include salaries, billing, claims adjustment, and other business overhead, such as activities relating to planning, regulating, and managing.

- -

Study after study shows that the U.S. has the highest healthcare administrative costs in the world. ✰

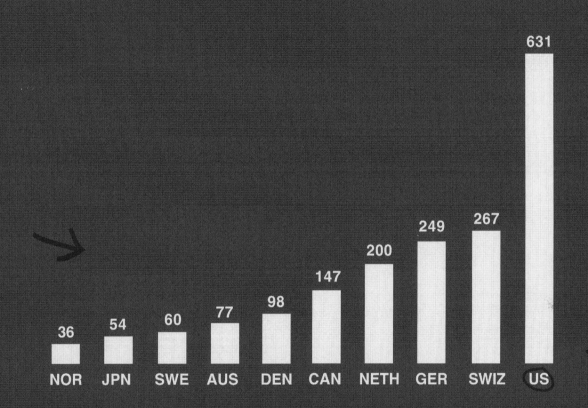

Spending On Health Insurance Adminstration Per Capita, 2012

In US Dollars & Adjusted for Differences in Costs of Living

Source: Organisation for Economic Co-operation and Development (OECD) Health Data. 2014

Counting Our Costs

Specifically with health insurance administration, we spend more than twice the administrative costs than our neighbor Canada does, according to researchers from The Commonweath Fund.

An often cited study of the costs of healthcare administration in the U.S. and Canada published in the New England Journal of Medicine in 2003 estimated that about 30% of American healthcare expenditures were the result of administration alone.

This was confirmed by a later study published in 2014, which found that hospital administrative costs accounted for 25.3% of total U.S. hospital expenditures, a percentage that is increasing and higher than any other country studied.

If that's not enough, another study published in 2018 in the Journal of American Medical Association regarding healthcare spending in the U.S. and other high-income countries concluded that administrative costs and pharmaceuticals appeared to be the major drivers of the difference in overall cost between the U.S. and other high-income countries.

Not only does having a private, insurance-based healthcare system increase the cost of administering healthcare in the U.S., our procedures also cost more. In 2012, Harvard published an analysis by the International Federation of Health Plans that showed variations in hospital procedure price by country.

The results are shocking, to say the least, with the U.S. having significantly higher costs for almost every procedure studied!

The average cost in the U.S. for a knee replacement is $25,637, which is almost $18,000 more than what the U.K. is charging at $7,883. In Australia, if you need your appendix removed, it will cost $5,467. In the U.S., the cost is $13,851.

Bypass surgery in Switzerland costs $17,729. In the U.S., a patient will be charged, on average, $73,420. A cesarean child birth will cost a U.S. patient $16,106 and a patient in Canada $5,980. A routine physician office visit costs about $95 for Americans but only $30 for the French. The average price of an MRI in the U.S. at $1,121 is significantly higher than in Spain at $235.

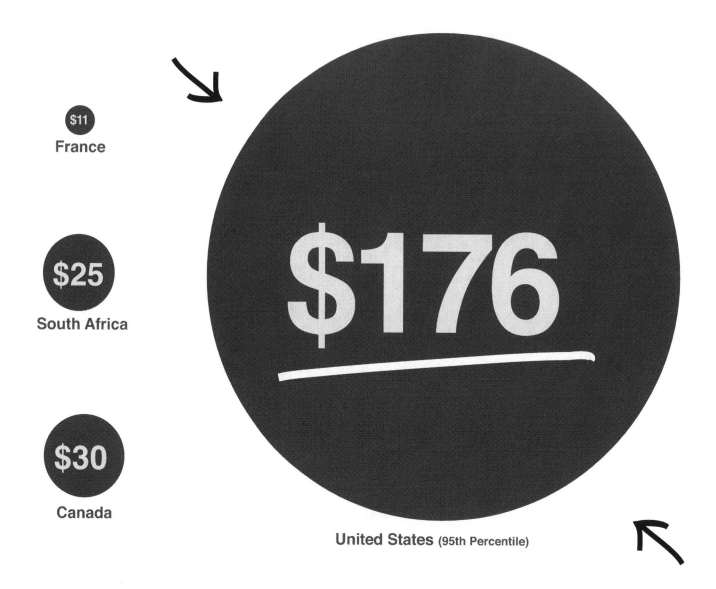

$11
France

$25
South Africa

$30
Canada

$176
United States (95th Percentile)

Routine Office Visit

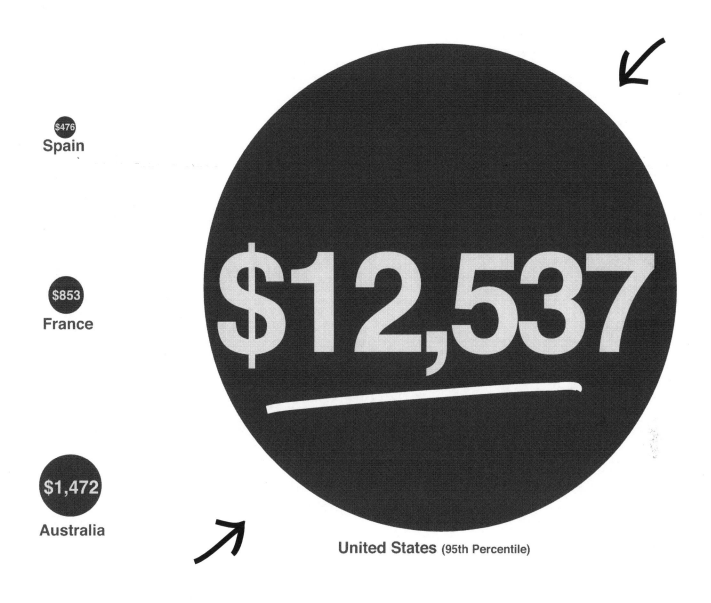

$476
Spain

$853
France

$1,472
Australia

$12,537

United States (95th Percentile)

Hospital Stay Per Day

Source: International Federation of Health Plans. 2012

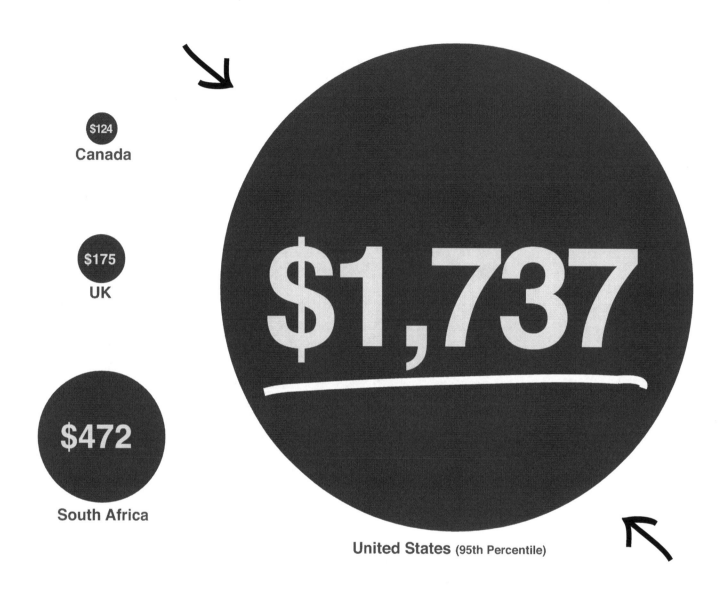

$124
Canada

$175
UK

$472
South Africa

$1,737
United States (95th Percentile)

Scanning and Imaging: CT Scan, Abdomen

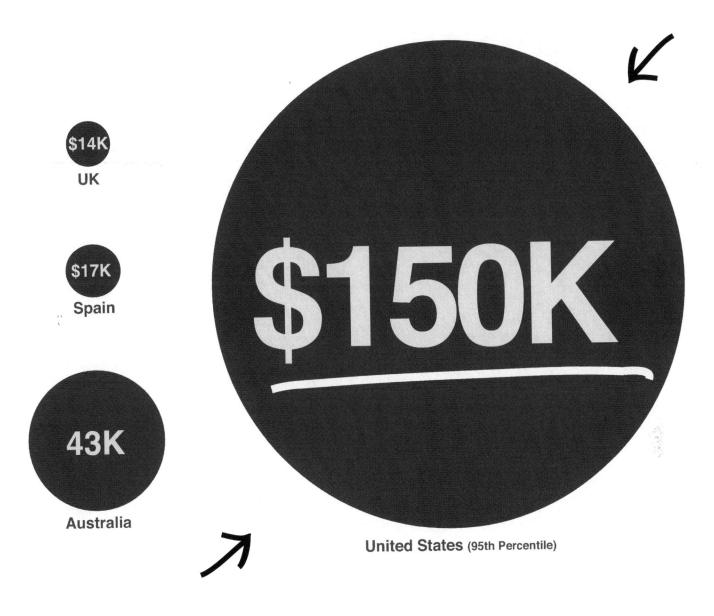

$14K
UK

$17K
Spain

43K
Australia

$150K

United States (95th Percentile)

Bypass Sugery

Source: International Federation of Health Plans. 2012

Counting Our Costs

Treating healthcare in the United States as a commodity also makes our pharmaceutical drugs cost more than in any other country—almost 3 times higher than in the United Kingdom in 2017.

In the U.S., many people with Multiple Sclerosis, a condition that affects the body's central nervous system, take Copaxone, which costs $3,900 each month. It's important to note here that this price is roughly the median monthly income for many Americans. In the Netherlands, the cost is $1,190 per month.

Truvada, prescribed to treat HIV/AIDS, is priced 89% higher than it is in the United Kingdom. The U.S. spent far more on pharmaceuticals than any other of the 35 OECD countries studied in 2018.

- -

No matter which study, chart, or table I find, it's a similar story. The United Stats has the world's most expensive healthcare system.

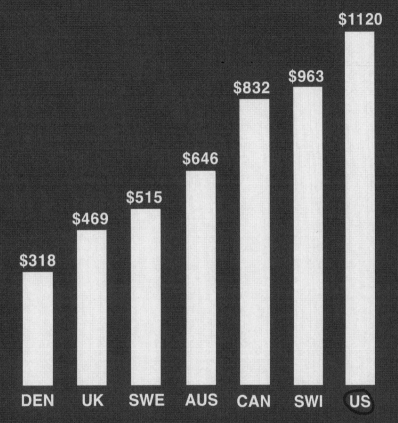

$1120

$963

$832

$646

$515

$469

$318

DEN UK SWE AUS CAN SWI US

Pharmaceutial Spending Per Capital, 2018*

2018 or Latest Available Data*

Source: Organisation for Economic Co-operation and Development (OECD) Health Data. 2019

Counting Our Costs

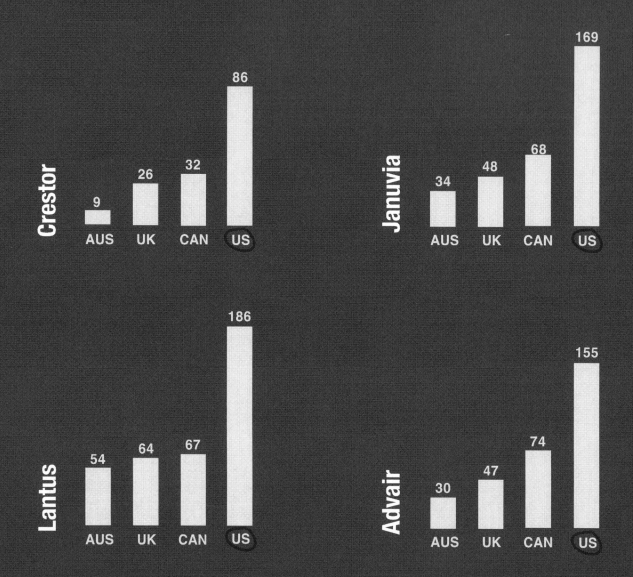

Monthly Price of Four Top Selling Prescription Drugs*
In U.S. Dollars*

Source: The Commonwealth Fund, 2017

Most often, we are not paying directly out of our own pocket but instead, indirectly through private insurance, which takes our money ahead of time to do so.

Regardless, we are paying more for healthcare whether we pay for it or someone else does it for us. We are trusting someone else to take care of paying our health claims.

We negotiate when we buy cars. We get upset when cable costs too much. Yet when it comes to healthcare, we don't question these costs.

These are the prices we are indirectly paying for, and comparable industrialized countries are providing the same products and services for a fraction of the price under some form of universal health coverage.

Americans are so accustomed to being removed from the payment process that we don't feel the direct pain. ✳

Chapter 3

A
Quality
Paradox

One would *think*...

that if we spend more money on something we are getting something better. There tends to be a stigma in America that we are getting something more; something that lasts longer, tastes better, has a cool feature—anything to provide more value and justify a higher cost.

This can go for anything: food, clothes, shoes, cars, and phones; if we spend more, we expect more. For example, clothes or shoes that last longer or cars that come with heated seats.

There are tangible differences between cotton and silk and a $5 steak versus a $40 steak.

Unfortunately, this concept is not the case within the healthcare industry. Is the real reason people do not question the high costs of healthcare because they think they are getting something better?

The bad news is that our healthcare system *does not* **provide any added** <u>values</u> **that come along with** *paying more.*

"The U.S healthcare system *consistently* ranks *last* in quality compared to other industrialized countries."

Source: The Commonwealth Fund & Center for Integrated Health Care

An important study titled *Mirror, Mirror* by The Commonwealth Fund collected information on a standardized set of metrics within health system performance and used data from several different reputable sources such as their own international surveys of patients and physicians, selected measures from OECD, WHO, and the European Observatory on Health Systems and Policies. It concluded that the U.S. ranks last in overall quality in comparison to ten other countries that are similar in wealth.

The U.S. fails every few years when they complete their research update.

The most recent update completed in 2017 shows the U.S. ranking last in several categories, including "health outcomes."

There are many ways to measure quality. I find one of the most useful ways is based on health outcomes and health status—*how people are living and their quality of life, because the goal of a well-functioning healthcare system is to ensure that people lead long, healthy, and productive lives.*

A Quality Paradox

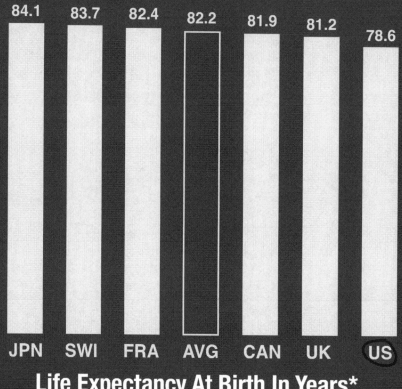

Life Expectancy At Birth In Years*

JPN	SWI	FRA	AVG	CAN	UK	US
84.1	83.7	82.4	82.2	81.9	81.2	78.6

2016 or Nearest Year*

Source: Kaiser Family Foundation Anaylsis of OECD Health Data. 2018

Life expectancy is one of the most often used health outcome indicators, and the U.S. ranks 27th in the world at 78.6 years. This is determined by social statistics such as living standards, lifestyle, access to education, access to quality health services, nutrition, sanitation, and housing—all relevant indicators of health status.

A Kaiser study in 2019 showed that the U.S. has the lowest life expectancy among comparable industrialized countries and has seen slower growth in life expectancy than comparable countries.

In fact, life expectancy in the U.S. has been dropping for several years, according to the CDC's National Center for Health Statistics.

The U.S has *lowest* life expectancy at birth among comparable countries.

A Quality Paradox

What's even more interesting is that there seems to be a significant connection between life expectancy and how much we spend on health in most countries. ⭐

- -

For developed countries, those increased health expenditures per person also increased longevity, but this is not the case for the U.S.

Again, *we are the lone-ranger in this data, set apart from the rest.*

It is certainly not a sign that we have the best healthcare system in the world if for double the resources our country uses, we still are not generating better health outcomes.

This indicates that more health spending isn't required to achieve better health results.

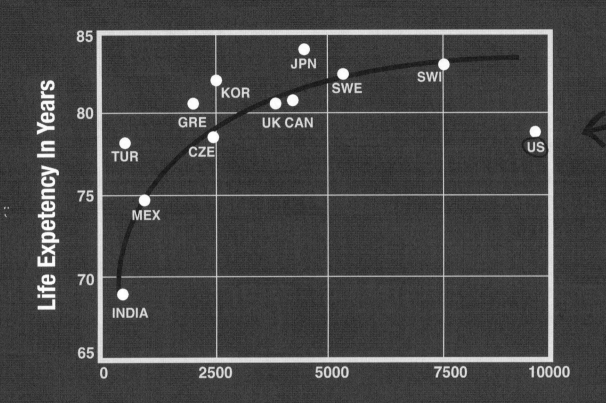

Source: Organisation for Economic Co-operation and Development (OECD) Health At A Glance. 2017

A Quality Paradox

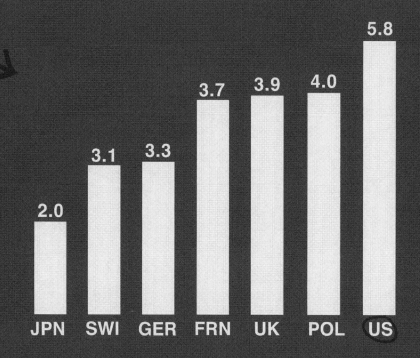

Infant Mortality Rate In Select OECD Countries, 2015*

Infant Deaths per 1,000 live births
*or nearest year

Source: Organisation for Economic Co-operation and Development (OECD) Health At A Glance. 2017

Another important health outcome indicator is infant mortality, the rate at which babies of less than one year of age die. This indicator reflects the cumulative effect of economic and social conditions, cultural lifestyles, and the characteristics and effectiveness of health systems. In alignment with the rest of the data already noted, the U.S. has a higher infant mortality rate than other comparable wealthy countries, according to OECD health data.

Further, the U.S. remains higher than the average of the 36 countries studied, especially for post-neonatal mortality (deaths after one month). A 2015 report from Save the Children: The State of the World's Mothers found the U.S. to have the highest first-day infant death rate in the industrialized world, ranking #33 worldwide, dropping from #30 in a previous analysis.

- -

It points out that in some U.S. cities, urban child survival gaps between rich and poor communities are greater than those found in developing countries.

A Quality Paradox

The U.S. also has the highest obesity rate in the world, and obesity is a health outcome influenced by a number of behavioral and environmental factors that contribute to a person's health and well-being.

These include access to nutritious food, exercise, and health education, as well as social determinants of health such as affordability and geographic location.

Social factors within the U.S. have created environments that place people, especially those who are socially vulnerable, more at risk of obesity.

While rates of obesity have consistently increased across the U.S. among people of all ethnic and racial groups, ages and genders, Black and Latino populations continue to have higher rates of obesity than whites and Asians, among both children and adults.

Many states in the south, such as Mississippi and Louisiana, have the highest obesity rates at approximately 37% of the population.

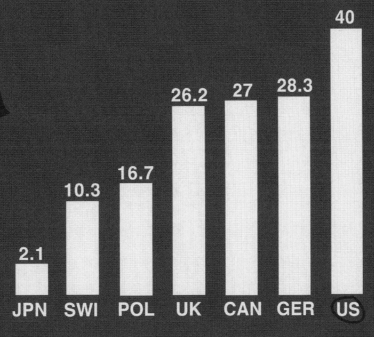

Obesity Rate in Adults, 2016*

As percent of total population (15 years & over)
Or Nearest Year*

Source: Organisation for Economic Co-operation and Development (OECD) Health Statistics. 2018

Listen !Up!

The long-term **rise** in **obesity** rates is a major public **health concern** because people who are overweight or obese are at greater risk of **poor health** throughout their lives. **Obesity** is a known risk factor for numerous health problems, including **diabetes, cardiovascular diseases, asthma, arthritis,** and some forms of **cancer.** It's also important to include **psychosocial problems** such as **depression, low self-esteem,** and **diminished quality of life** as a result from being **overweight.**

A Quality Paradox

Beyond obesity and life expectancy as health outcome indicators, the safety of patients when they are using the system is also a measure for determining a quality and well-functioning healthcare system. According to a handful of studies, including the British Medical Journal, Journal of Patient Safety, and data from the Centers for Disease Control (CDC), the third leading cause of death in the U.S. after heart disease and cancer is medical errors.

Undetected diagnostic errors and medical mistakes can result in someone's death, which the researchers now say translates to 9.5% of all deaths each year in the U.S. This provides another reason as to why the U.S. ranks so low in quality in numerous studies, because quality is an output of how safe and effective a health system functions.

Medical errors signify a moral, professional, and public health *dilemma.*

"**Medical errors—** *third* **leading cause of death in the U.S.**"

Source: Journal of Patient Safety & British Medical Journal

A Quality Paradox

Healthcare in the U.S. continues to harm an unacceptable number of patients. Every year, 1 in 20 Americans receiving outpatient care are misdiagnosed due to fraud or personal failure of the physician in a study done by the National Academy of Sciences in 2015.

Misdiagnosis, in whichever form, can result in serious complications, including infection and even death. In fact, in another study published in the Journal of Patient Safety, each year, between 210,000 and 440,000 patients suffer some type of preventable harm while they are in the hospital that contributes to their death.

This amounts to 1,000 or more deaths per day due to hospital medical errors and infections.

Researchers from these studies caution that most medical errors aren't due to inherently bad physicians; rather, most errors represent systemic problems, including poorly coordinated care, fragmented insurance networks, the absence of safety nets, inappropriate incentives, and more.

Diagnostic mistakes are just one type of error that occurs in healthcare. Providers of care often make horrendous errors, such as treating the wrong patient, leaving behind surgical tools in a person after surgery, or operating on the wrong body part.

Other examples of potentially fatal medical errors that are all too common include: air bubbles in your blood after a chest tube is removed, mix-ups involving medical tubing, incorrect medication dosing, and hospital-acquired infections. All of which are preventable.

The concept of "mortality amenable to health care" as an indicator of how effectively healthcare is being delivered has been studied several times in the past.

- -

Amenable translates to preventable and avoidable. In a 2014 study, the U.S. had the highest mortality amenable to health care at 112 deaths per 100,000 people. ✯

A Quality Paradox

Another health outcome indicator that indicates poor quality, widely accepted by public health advocates, is the rate of readmissions to a hospital.

Readmission is commonly defined as a patient having been discharged from a hospital and then being admitted again within a specified time interval, usually within 30 days.

Preventing readmissions has the potential to greatly improve both the quality of life for patients and the financial well-being of our healthcare system.

One study commissioned by the Alliance for Home Health Quality and Innovation (AHHQI) finds that, specific to Medicare patients, a single preventable return trip to the hospital more than doubles the cost of care.

Although not all readmissions can be prevented, research shows that there are strategies that hospitals can apply to avoid many of their readmissions, such as telephone calls, house visits, telemonitoring, and changes to hospital procedures.

There is good news here; readmission rates are dropping, and that is because they have been targeted as a high priority for U.S. healthcare reform efforts. The Hospital Readmissions Reduction Program, which was a part of the Affordable Care Act (ACA), applied financial penalties to hospitals that have excess readmission rates for targeted conditions, such as heart attack, knee replacements, and pneumonia. Under the law, hospitals can incur a penalty of up to 3% of their Medicare payments.

In 2018, Medicare fined 2,599 hospitals for high readmission rates under this legislation with New Jersey, West Virginia, and Delaware having the highest percentage of hospitals in their states penalized.

Several different studies have analyzed data from over 3,000 hospitals from 2007 to 2018 and found that readmission rates are continuously declining after holding steady for several years.

This is because money has a big influence on changing behaviors and has forced providers to begin taking quality seriously.

A Quality Paradox

A *considerable* amount of evidence demonstrates the <u>numerous</u> ways the transition out of the hospital and into the next place of care can be inconsistent, *unsafe,* rushed, confusing, and *ineffective.*

These attributes lead to patients coming back to the hospital to be readmitted.

- -

For example, readmission interviews found that a 46-year-old, Spanish-speaking-only female with breast cancer was hospitalized six times and visited the emergency department three times in one year.

The patient received instructions in English, and her twelve-year-old daughter was asked to translate. The patient had a poor understanding of prescription instructions in English, and her twelve-year-old daughter was asked to translate. The patient had a poor understanding of prescription instructions. The hospital could have used interpreter services to confirm understanding and clarify any questions.

Another example details a 24-year-old female with HIV/AIDS, hospitalized eight times and visited the emergency department twice in one year. They were first hospitalized for pneumonia, then readmitted eight days later for pneumonia. When asked how the hospital could have helped her prepare to leave the hospital, she said, "Make all appointments before I leave the hospital." It was clear this patient needed assistance navigating the healthcare system.

Other patient and clinical factors that predict readmission have been determined by research and includes the quality of inpatient care and surgical complications.

A Quality Paradox

A study published in the New England Journal of Medicine has shown that nearly one in seven patients hospitalized for a major surgical procedure is readmitted to the hospital within 30 days after discharge. Surgical complications and hospital readmissions shortly after discharge have plagued inpatient healthcare for a long time, causing higher costs and adverse health events for patients. Complications include any minor or major deviations from the normal, post-surgery recovery process. Possible complications include: fever and infection, pain, foreign objects left behind, and pulmonary issues, amongst many others. A Surgeon Dashboard was developed by ProPublica researchers in 2015 that calculated death and complication rates for surgeons performing one of eight elective procedures in Medicare. Their output was a database to be used as a resource for patients to learn more about a surgeon before their operation.

The analysis notes that although conventional wisdom tells patients to simply choose a reputable hospital when they need surgery, they found that even within "good" hospitals, performance between surgeons can vary significantly, and half of all hospitals in America have surgeons with low and high complication rates.

The following is an example of a result from their database on Methodist Stone Oak Hospital in San Antonio, Texas. This is a great example of why there are penalties for readmissions, as none of the surgeons at this hospital has a low complication rate. You may want to seek another hospital or discuss complication rates in more detail with a surgeon from that hospital if you are planning to have knee or gallbladder surgery. Thankfully for patients that need these surgeries, the surgeon's name appears when you hover your mouse over the tick mark on the website.

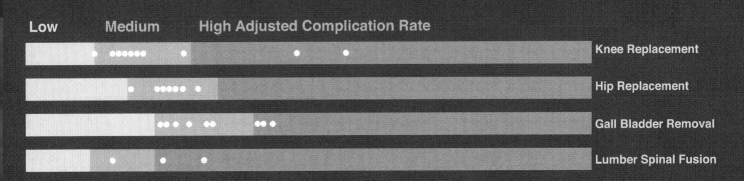

Low   Medium   High Adjusted Complication Rate

Knee Replacement

Hip Replacement

Gall Bladder Removal

Lumber Spinal Fusion

How Surgeons At Methodist Stone Oak Hospital Perform By Procedure

• Indicates a particular surgeon

So, how did we get to having such a *dysfunctional* healthcare system with *high* costs and *low* quality?

In the U.S., the roots of healthcare were not in business but instead, as social movements. Institutions began as a way to care for the sick and injured while the wealthy received care at home from physicians. Boston opened the first general hospital in 1864 for the non-wealthy with an interest in protecting the community from the spread of contagious diseases.

The motivation was service, not profit.

In 1946, the Hill-Burton Act was created to provide funding to meet the needs of war victims as the current system was not able to keep up; facilities needed to be upgraded, new buildings needed to be built, and more supplies were needed. The government and wealthy investors stepped in to provide, which increased the need for a more business-centered approach, due to the red-tape of regulation and investment

Now, we treat healthcare as a commodity and not a right, which has led to poor social responsibility and fiscal irresponsibility, very far away from its roots as a social service.

Part 2

Why Does Not Ｗant Know ―

The System You To ?

Before starting, please take five minutes to reflect upon the quote on the following page. Feel free to use the space provided below to write, draw or sketch anything that comes to your mind.

↓

"All men make mistakes**, but a** good **man yields when he** knows **his course is wrong, and** repairs **the evil. The only crime is** pride**."**
— Sophocles

↑

Chapter 4

Back
To
Ethics

Although it *isn't* certain where this quote comes from...

quoted by many as being from Frank Outlaw or Charles Reade, it does sum up quite well where our personal ethics and morals come from. I have shared it with my students at the beginning of every healthcare ethics course I've taught:

 "Watch your thoughts, they become words;
watch your words, they become actions;
watch your actions, they become habits;
watch your habits, they become character;
watch your character, for it becomes your destiny."

- -

Essentially, what we think about ultimately determines our ethics and develops our character.

The types of thoughts that we harbor in our minds and the people, media, and books that we engage with influence what we think about. These thoughts develop implicit biases, which refer to the attitudes or stereotypes that affect our actions in an unconscious manner. Every moment our brains process incredible amounts of information. This processing allows us to make decisions and take action. The majority of which goes on behind the scenes.

Writer and blogger Ian Welsh says that "*morals are how you treat people you know and ethics are how you treat people you don't know*." These quotes are both powerful ways to frame the idea of morals and how we interact with society. We are not born with a character; therefore, our morals are developed and evolve as life happens. Every experience and interaction we have contributes to the bottom line of what our morals are. The personal values that we develop as a result of living life creates the foundation for making decisions, guiding behavior, and establishing priorities.

This diversity gives rise to ethical dilemmas, which are situations where people disagree, and there are many opportunities for this in healthcare.

Back To Ethics

Twentieth century philosopher Lawrence Kohlberg devised a theory about how one becomes an ethical person. He called it Stages of Moral Development and concluded that people must go through one stage of development at a time before moving on to the next, and we move through six stages as we find solutions to the challenges we face in life.

Therefore, some people are unable to make certain decisions because of their ethical maturity. Even though someone is an adult physically, they can be morally immature due to the challenges they've been through and how they responded to them.

The first two stages in Kohlberg's theory are called Premoral or before moral reasoning. It's all about you. Your decisions are centered on yourself, and you make them to avoid punishment and/or to obtain personal rewards. It's about selfishness, and people are valued at how useful they are to you.

However, although this is common in children, some adults still fit this category.

The next stages are **Externally Controlled Morals** or rules of society and culture. Decisions are made to please people and to obey laws. People make moral decisions because they want to be seen as good people, good employees, good friends, good spouses, good students. Most people remain on these levels. The last stages are called **Principled Morals** or rules of a higher authority. These include making decisions with the thought that everyone is entitled to common rights.

A respect for yourself and tolerance for others requires complex thinking about how you relate with others going beyond what is law. This is believing that all humans have worth and value regardless of their social status.

For example, segregation was legal at one time; however, it was unethical and violated a higher law.

- -

Only 25% of the population *actually* gets to these last levels of highest ethical development and maturity.

Would you prioritize life? What would — self? For your loved

According to the Associated Press, a Brookdale Senior Residence facility worker, who —
(CPR) to Lorraine Bayless, an 87-year-old woman who collapsed in the facility's dining —

Although the nurse called 911 and the dispatcher urged her to start CPR or to find —
was no Do Not Resuscitate (DNR) directive in place. Shortly after this report, Brookdale —
patcher's directions was a mistaken interpretation of the policy. How you would act in —

Sorry, your *life* is aga

Write your response here:

your **job** or a **human**

-you *want* for your-

ones?

Ethics Case Study - Waiting to Die
Is it Healthcare or a Corporate Dystopia?

▶ identified herself as a nurse, refused to administer cardiopulmonary resuscitation
▶ hall. "It was against company policy."

someone who was willing to do so, the nurse refused. The press reported that there
⟶ Senior Living issued a statement saying the employee's failure to heed a 911 dis-
▶ this instance makes a big distinction about your morals and values.

---

inst *company* policy.

If our experience helps shape our morals, then we need experiences. People without kids do not truly understand people who have kids. The same goes for people with pets or people who have lost a child to gun violence. How can we truly feel empathy for somebody in a certain situation until we experience it on our own? Consider the following:

Can people who have never been uninsured have empathy for people who have no insurance? Can a politician that has never been without insurance advocate for a system that includes all? Will the Chief Executive Officer (CEO) of an insurance company make decisions to reduce premiums if she has never suffered personal bankruptcy due to health care expenses? Can a man that has never been sexually advanced, groped, molested, or raped develop policies effectively for a woman who has?

Yes, it is possible. People with higher ethical maturity levels have the ability to do these things.

These types of people, I argue, are the kind of leaders we need making decisions in healthcare.

If one wants to buy a Mercedes, they can go to a car dealer, pick a color, arrange financing, and have a new car. If one can't afford to buy a Mercedes, then maybe they will leave the Mercedes dealer and pursue a Ford Focus or decide to just stick with riding the bus. Either way, you, the consumer, are in charge of that purchase. Mercedes isn't responsible or under obligation if one cannot secure financing or afford the car with cash. The luxury car maker has no ethical duty to the consumer.

Although healthcare is a business, too, it has very different financial obligations than other industries within our economy. People do not want to purchase cancer treatments, chronic disease remedies, asthma inhalers, or request hip surgery. In the United States, healthcare consumers are not in control of most health-related purchases outside of the retail market because insurance companies make most health-related decisions for them. Health consumers know premiums, deductibles, and co-payments, which are the entry fees into the U.S. healthcare system. Their choice and role in purchasing is minimal. As a result, we cannot treat healthcare like any other industry in the free market.

A healthcare system cannot function *without* the boundaries of duty and obligation like Mercedes *can*.

However, the reality for Americans is that we are operating outside of those boundaries in a system without duty to the human being. American healthcare is a commodity treated like any other industry within the market economy and is not managed like a human right. Because someone else takes care of our limited healthcare dollars, using them must be done in a responsible way. The balance of profit and social justice is a true dilemma in our healthcare system, but it is not impossible to balance that scale. If leaders of an organization are motivated by money, it can deter the mission of caring for the sick and injured, promoting prevention, and keeping people healthy and happy. Fiscal responsibility is a duty to be responsible and accountable with money, especially someone else's, and is a marriage of numbers and values.

Therefore, an organization's financial statement is their ethical statement. ✶

This is because what an organization prioritizes and spends their money on defines what's important to them.

One of the biggest issues we have in the U.S. healthcare system is not not having enough money for healthcare, but it is how that money is spent. Not only do health consumers spend a substantial amount of money by way of insurance premiums but also, in taxes. There are a lot of healthcare dollars being spent right now; it's how we spend them that determines what's important to us.

- -

Check out the salaries on the next set of pages of top health industry executives, and consider what their organizations prioritize and what their values are.

CEO		COMPANY
Michael Neidorff	OF	**Centene**
Bruce Broussard	OF	**Humana**
Mark Bertolini	OF	**Aetna**
David Cordani	OF	**Cigna**
David Wichmann	OF	**UHG***
Joseph Swedish	OF	**Wellpoint**
Allen Wise	OF	**Covetry**
Jay Gallert	OF	**Health Net**
Paula Steiner	OF	**HCSC***

*UnitedHealth Group

*Healthcare Service Corporation

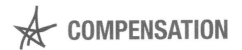 **COMPENSATION**

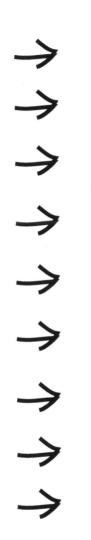

$25,000,000

$20,000,000

$19,000,000

$18,000,000

$17,000,000

$17,000,000

$15,000,000

$12,000,000

$6,000,000

Source: Becker's Hospital Review, Bloomberg, and Equiliar. CEO salaries of health insurance companies, 2018 or latest (some data 2017). Data includes salary, stock options exercised/or granted, and bonuses.

CEO		COMPANY
Anthony Tersigni	OF	**Ascension Health**
Michael Dowling	OF	**Norwell Health**
Daniel Evans	OF	**IU Health**
James Skogsberg	OF	**Advocate Health**
Steven Aslchuler	OF	**CH of Philly**
Randall O'Donnell	OF	**CMH of Kansas***
John Koster	OF	**Providence**
Judith Persichilli	OF	**Trinity Health**
Dean Harrison	OF	**NWMH***

*Childrens Mercy Hospital of Kansas

*Nortwestern Memorial Hopsital of IllinoiS

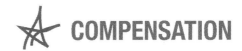 **COMPENSATION**

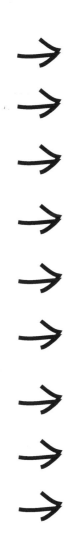

$18,000,000

$10,000,000

$8,000,000

$8,000,000

$6,000,000

$6,000,000

$6,000,000

$5,000,000

$5,000,000

Source: Becker's Hospital Review, Bloomberg, and Equiliar. CEO salaries of health insurance companies, 2018 or latest (some data 2017). Data includes salary, stock options exercised/or granted, and bonuses.

CEO		COMPANY
Martine Rothblatt	OF	**United Therapeutics**
Alex Gorsky	OF	**Johnson & Johnson**
Ian Read	OF	**Pfizer**
Lamberto Andreotti	OF	**Bristol-Meyers S.**
John Hammergren	OF	**McKesson Corp**
John Martin	OF	**Gilead**
Heather Bresch	OF	**Mylan**
Larry Merlo	OF	**CVS Health Corp**
George Barret	OF	**Cardinal Health**

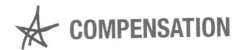 **COMPENSATION**

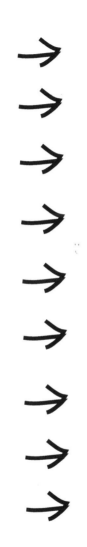

$37,000,000

$30,000,000

$28,000,000

$19,000,000

$18,000,000

$15,000,000

$13,000,000

$12,000,000

$11,000,000

Source: Becker's Hospital Review, Bloomberg, and Equiliar. CEO salaries of health insurance companies, 2018 or latest (some data 2017). Data includes salary, stock options exercised/or granted, and bonuses.

Chapter 5

Fiscal

Irresponsibillity

Nearly *all* large healthcare organizations make their top executives *extremely* rich, a perverse <u>incentive</u> to *profit* off the *sick.*

Sarah Anderson, Global Economy Director at the Institute for Policy Studies, said,

"If executives are loaded up with stock options and other types of equity-based pay, they have a personal incentive to boost share prices by whatever means necessary."

One top earner is CEO Martine Rothblatt of the pharmaceutical company United Therapeutics. She took home $37 million in 2018.

United Therapeutics manufactures drugs to treat high blood pressure and for pediatrics with high-risk cancers.

For comparison purposes, Seema Verma, the administrator who oversees Medicaid and Medicare, is given a $165,000 salary, paid for by tax dollars.

If she was getting paid $5 million from our tax money, there would be upheaval about how our tax money is spent.

- -

How come we don't question *how* our healthcare dollars are *spent*?

Health **insurance** →

raising (our) premiums →

collect millions →

meanwhile, →

borrowing $88 billion →

healthcare **expenses,** →

a ~~medical treatment~~ →

leaders are **are** comfortable

~~every~~ year as they

of dollars in **salary;**

Americans are

annually to **pay** for their

and **one in four** skipped

because of cost.

Source: 2019 Gallup Poll

Where do *you* think these executives <u>fall</u> within Kohlberg's ethical maturity levels?

In the current environment of 30 million people being uninsured and millions of others having high deductibles they can't afford, do you think it's acceptable for these types of compensations? Is it justified or fair that health CEO's have taken home 11% more of our money on average every year since 2010, according to an Axios analysis? What are the priorities of these executives when they take such high salaries? Is this fiscally responsible with our limited shared resources? Welcome to the executive compensation problem that exists in the United States. Other countries don't seem to have the same CEO compensation problem that we do.

How big of an ego does the U.S. have?

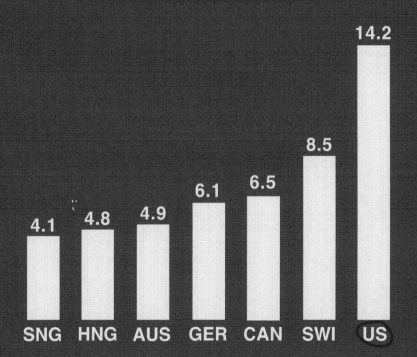

Average Annual CEO Compensation Worldwide by Country, 2017

In Millions of U.S Dollars

Source: Bloomberg

Fiscal Irresponsibility

As a response to the economic crisis of our recent past and in an effort to avoid future widespread financial collapse, the Dodd-Frank Wall Street Reform and Consumer Protection Act was signed into law in 2010.

The law was designed to increase transparency in executive compensation by requiring publicly traded companies to publish CEO pay figures, median worker pay, and the ratio between CEO and median worker pay. This data began to be shared in 2017 for the first time.

It was found that for several years in a row, healthcare executives led the S&P 500 in terms of total compensation, surpassing industries such as energy, technology, and finance, and CEO pay remains high, relative to the pay of typical workers.

In 2018, health insurance company Humana had their CEO making 344 times more than their typical worker, and Universal Health Services, a national hospital management company, led the results with a ratio at 541:1.

A lower ratio indicates companies dedicated to creating high-wage jobs and investing in their employees instead of a winner-take-all attitude where executives reap the biggest share of compensation.

These types of pay gaps help to fuel the extreme inequality that exists in the United States. The typical CEO in the healthcare system made $16.1 million in 2018.

To put that into perspective, this is equivalent to *200* employees making an annual salary of *$80,500*.

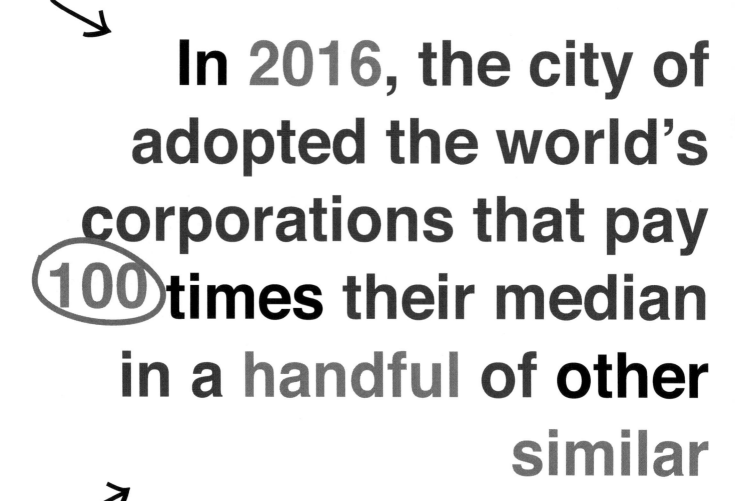

In 2016, **the city of adopted the world's corporations that pay** 100 **times their median in a** handful **of other** similar

Portland, Oregon first tax penalty on their CEO more than worker pay. Lawmakers states are considering legislation.

Kohlberg's Stages of Moral Development theory notes that it is possible...

for people to be unable to make certain decisions due to ethical maturity. This provides a possible explanation for how healthcare executives can take home salaries of multi-millions of dollars amidst all the challenges the healthcare system currently faces. People are unable to afford a necessary surgery, procedure, or medication because their deductibles are too high; every six minutes a patient dies in an American hospital from a hospital-acquired infection. Preventable hospital errors persist as the number three killer in the U.S.—third only to heart disease and cancer, and on average, a hospital patient is subject to one medication error per day.

Large corporations and CEOs will argue that these wages are necessary to attract the best and brightest executives to the healthcare industry.

How is it that our executive healthcare leaders think they deserve such pay when our system is in shambles? Refer back to part one of this book. For most other people in the corporate world, bonuses and raises are based on performance and hitting targets and goals. I can't imagine we are hitting targets and goals with the current state of our healthcare system. Or maybe the targets and goals should change? CEO Wayne Smith of Community Health Systems received $16 million in total compensation, yet recently settled a lawsuit alleging false billing and kickback allegations, both federal crimes. If our system was booming with better health outcomes, affordable coverage, less fraud, and no uninsured, then perhaps it would be justified to have executives taking such high pays. Further, if we treat healthcare as a right or, like most countries do, as any other public service like the library or police, then our current system functions without morals or pre-moral stage one-two.

If leaders in healthcare had a stage five or six ethical maturity level (principled morals of a higher authority), do you think they would take salaries such as these? It is hard to argue that these executive leaders are ethically mature.

Did You

?

Know?

Babbit Municipalities Inc., a Chicago based benefits administrator for labor unions, developed a class action lawsuit against Health Care Service Corporation (HCSC) alleging the company has not upheld its nonprofit mission by giving their executive team $16 million in compensation in 2012. The suit argues that the $100 million that was paid out in bonuses to ten top executives between 2011 and 2013 should have been given back to health plan members in rebates or in lower future premiums.

Fiscal Irresponsibility

Healthcare isn't Pepsi, Coach, Kellogg, Hilton, Koehler, or Mercedes. People don't need to drink Pepsi, wear Coach bags, eat corn flakes, or stay at hotels to survive, but they do need access to healthcare for optimal health and wellness. Leaders in healthcare must have different values than leaders in other industries within the shared economy because of this striking truth.

To put this into perspective, let's examine the scenarios of CEOs taking a pay cut:

1. Randall O'Donnell is the CEO at Children's Mercy Hospital in Kansas City, Missouri and makes $6 million a year. How many nurses could the hospital hire if Randall only made $1 million a year and put the other $5M toward the nurse shortage to increase the quality of patient care? According to indeed.com, the average nurse's annual salary is $65,000 a year in Kansas City, MO; simplyhired.com puts it at $49,000, and ehow.com notes the average registered nurse salary at $55,150. The median of them is $55,150. If we assume $65,000 as an average "all-in" cost for a nurse, how many nurses, with a cost of $65,000 annually, could be hired for $5 million? At least seventy-five more nurses could be employed, if the hospital CEO didn't make $6 million annually.

2. Former Blue Cross Blue Shield of Illinois CEO Patricia Hemingway-Hall received $16 million in compensation, plus a $15 million bonus, totaling $31 million in 2012. In the year before, they laid off almost one hundred people. Reducing her pay to $1 million would bring how many people back to work? If we generously used an average all-in salary of $65,000, we could bring back all one hundred people and have as much as $20 million left over to reduce deductibles for individual plans in the state marketplaces.

The opportunities are endless for what healthcare executives can do with our healthcare dollars instead of high salaries for themselves and the rest of their executive team: lowering of deductibles and copayments, adding additional coverage such as functional medicine, holistic practitioners, and massage therapy, or increases in salaries for workers. Organizations are willing to give these services up when they take on large, multi-million-dollar salaries for their executive teams. Again, an organization's financial statement is their ethics statement.

Do you think they are acting with social and fiscal responsibility?

→ Exercise! What's Your **Priority?** ←

Consider you are on the management team at a small community hospital and planning your upcoming year's budget. You have 100 healthcare resources (money, people, technology). Decide what gets how much of these resources by putting numbers in the boxes and continually adding up the running total until you reach 100. Distribute as you feel ethically fit. Do your best to be good stewards of the limited financial resources and act with social and fiscal responsibility to the best of your ability. Remember that an organization's financial statement is their ethics statement.

☐ **Staff Development Program** + ☐ **Community Wellness Program** = _____ /100

↓

☐ **Mental Health Clinic** + ☐ **Two ER Patients Without Insurance** = _____ /100

↓

☐ **Salaries For Executive Team** + ☐ **Salaries For Clinical Staff** = _____ /100

↓

☐ **Laboratory Equipment Servicing** + ☐ **Cancer Patient Needing Radiation Treatment** = _____ /100

For pharmaceutical companies specifically, where executive compensation is *higher* than in most healthcare sectors, consumers do not *directly* feel the *pain* of the high costs of prescription drugs.

This is because the costs are in co-pays, which are set fees we can expect. The high costs of their drugs are filtered through the system and hidden as higher premiums and deductibles because our insurance companies pay the rest of the bill for us with our premium dollars.

We are not only paying for the drug itself but also, supporting a $66 million salary for its CEO. In 2017, healthcare reporter Bob Herman published an analysis of the salaries of over 100 CEO's of 70 of the largest U.S. healthcare companies based on corporate financial filings.

Cumulatively, these CEO's have earned $9.8 billion since 2010. Imagine the magnitude of those dollars and how they could be spent differently within our system. The Institute for Policy Studies notes that $75 million is the equivalent of the cost of dental insurance for 250,000 Americans or the average annual health insurance plan deductible for 24,000 people. That is just a small fraction of that $9.8 billion.

Even more, consider the cumulative cost of the rest of the c-suite that get similar salaries: CFO, CEO, COO, CIO. An analysis done by Modern Healthcare noted that one company alone, Health Care Service Corp., the Blue Cross and Blue Shield insurer in five states, paid their top ten executives, cumulatively, $56.7 million in 2015.

Chapter 6

Motivated
By Money

There are several familiar *guiding principles* of healthcare ethics such as doing no harm, preserving life, being discreet, upholding justice, and respecting autonomy.

Healthcare leaders will never be given enough resources to satisfy all the demands placed upon them by a community, but they can turn to the guiding principle of justice to help them distribute their yearly budgets ethically.

Justice refers to fairness and equality and stems from a rather simple yet complex ethical concept called the Philosophy of Individual Worth.

It is a duty and moral obligation for healthcare systems to give the same treatment to everyone, regardless of one's circumstances.

Leaders in healthcare have a *duty* to go beyond personal feelings and honor an individual's worth. We want the same don't we—for people to *respect* our needs and what we want and believe?

But this is hard to do, and as a result, leaders in healthcare must have this skill, which I argue is only possible by some with higher ethical maturity.

What does the moral duty of tolerance look like in healthcare?

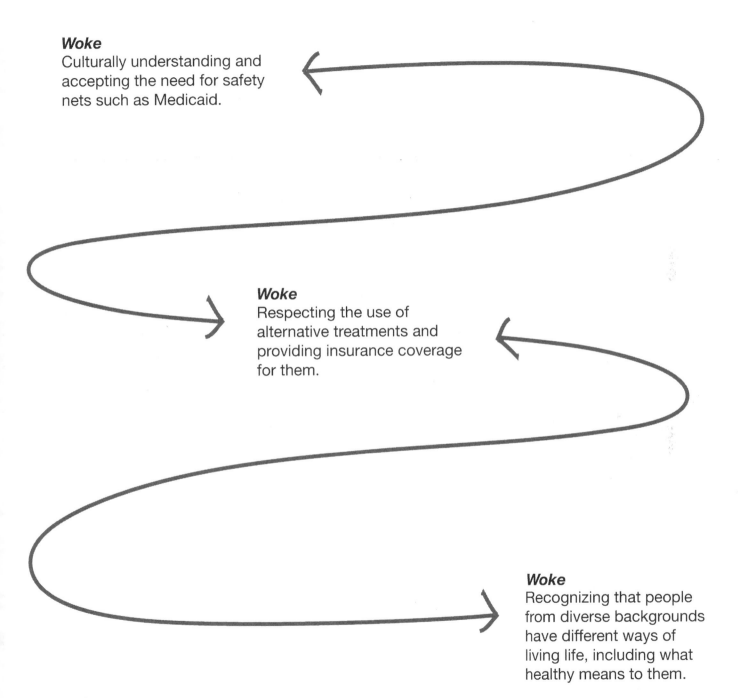

Woke
Culturally understanding and accepting the need for safety nets such as Medicaid.

Woke
Respecting the use of alternative treatments and providing insurance coverage for them.

Woke
Recognizing that people from diverse backgrounds have different ways of living life, including what healthy means to them.

Motivated By Money

Justice is also the fair distribution of benefits offered by a society and includes the fair distribution of its burdens, as well. The problem the U.S. has with its uninsured is a failure of the ethical principle of distributive justice, the concept of justice and equality before the law is embedded within societies all over the world. A Spanish proverb states that "a rule isn't unfair if it applies to everyone," and a founding principle of the United States is "equal justice under law," which is the caption on the facade of the Federal Supreme Court building.

Society suffers injustice when not everyone gets to share the benefits and when distributions of resources are not equal. In healthcare, this creates an environment where health equity is compromised, and health disparities shade society with injustice, which is the unfortunate reality in the United States.

Because we live in a healthcare system where someone else takes care of our healthcare dollars, the concept of good financial stewardship and the duty to be fiscally responsible with limited healthcare resources is supported by the ethical principle of justice.

Members of racial and ethnic *minorities* **are less likely to receive preventive health services, more likely to be uninsured, often receive lower-quality care, and have** *worse* **health outcomes for many conditions in comparison to whites.**

Motivated By Money

Award-winning 20th century philosopher John Rawls was interested in what makes a just and moral society. He formulized a hypothetical theory where people are equal to each other, and all humans have worth in the Original Position, and if we take a Veil of Ignorance with each other, a social contract would develop that secures basic rights for everyone and protects those in all positions of society.

His theory goes on to say that the advantaged have a responsibility to the disadvantaged. Those that are disadvantaged could include those in poverty, those with chronic diseases that affect quality of life, the disabled, etc.

Therefore, in the end, it is in our ultimate best interest to do this because everyone has the potential to be in the lesser position (loss of job, health, etc.) Rawl developed these theories during the Great Depression, when people's lives regularly changed overnight. John Rawls said:

"A just society is a society that if you knew everything about it, you'd be willing to enter it in a random place."

Consider that powerful thought: are you willing to be born into a low-income, black family in Philadelphia or Chicago? Statistically, this population has the highest rate of health disparities in the country, and as a result, end up in unhealthy situations that produce another statistic: highest homicide rate in the country.

At the core of Rawls theory is that no matter what our circumstance, environment, or influence, we are human, and all human interests must be observed to truly live in a moral, ethical, and just society. This is not what our reality is today, especially not in our healthcare system.

And although I like the concept of having a "veil of ignorance," I believe our societal issues can't be solved by ignoring characteristics but instead—acceptance of them. A just society comes from tolerance and not from direct ignorance. If we want people to be tolerant of our ideals, we must be tolerant of others.

This is why the balancing scales are often the symbol used for justice. Only one set of ideals getting priority does not work.

Can the CEO of a pharmaceutical company ~~prioritize~~ opioid addiction as a top concern if they are making a profit from opioids?

Can specialty physicians prioritize preventative health, physicals, and early screenings if they are doctors for people who are sick?

How can **providers** ~~prioritize~~ the **welfare** of their patients if **compensation** is <u>tied</u> to how many **services** they provide?

Motivated By Money

Just as healthcare leaders reduce the number of nurses on the floor that care for patients in order to save healthcare dollars, maybe we should consider eliminating a few million dollars of executive pay instead. What do you think will positively impact patients more: fewer nurses or less executive pay?

According to a study published in the Journal of the American Medical Association, there is no link between CEO pay and hospital quality indicators, such as readmission rates, mortality rates, or community outreach programs. In other words, a highly paid CEO will not necessarily increase the performance of a hospital and the outcomes of patients.

It's unsettling that CEO's at hospitals with high mortality rates are being paid just as much, or sometimes more, as those at hospitals with lower rates of mortality. Physician compensation is increasingly being tied to quality measures, and I argue that healthcare executives should be treated the same given that they have a fiduciary and ethical responsibility to represent the welfare of the community in which they serve.

An analysis by Kaiser Health News found that it was more common for executive bonuses to be tied to boosting volume rather than increasing quality, which unfortunately, creates an environment where the incentive is to keep people returning to the hospital, not preventing them from needing to be readmitted.

Surgeon Paul Ruggieri candidly writes about an encounter with a patient referred for removal of gallstones in his book, *The Cost of Cutting: A Surgeon Reveals The Truth Behind A Multibillion-Dollar Industry,*

"For a brief moment—and this is *difficult* to admit—I found myself tempted to schedule the surgery. A completely *unnecessary* surgery."

I *believe* wholeheartedly that ethically mature leaders in healthcare exist...

and are capable of making major healthcare business decisions without the multi-million-dollar salary to prove their worth and competency. The present chaos that exists within our healthcare system shows that the current model of excessive executive compensation is not working and immoral.

With that, I am calling for policymakers, taxpayers, and health consumers to consider new public policy to tackle the injustice of excessive executive pay that exists in the American healthcare system.

- -

I am proposing a professional consideration of placing caps and limits on executive compensation in these fields. ⭐

This is argued based on the fact that healthcare is something every human needs and is an industry that all are born into, live in, and die in; it simply cannot be employed in the same manner as a company that sells running shoes.

The recommended process for determining the appropriate compensation, usually, is to conduct a review of what similarly-sized organizations in the same geography offer their senior leaders.

However, since healthcare is not like any other industry due to its ethical duties and obligations, the same process simply cannot apply.

A new way of calculating executive compensation must be developed, so precious and limited healthcare resources can be distributed fairly and used effectively.

We must begin to champion efforts for fiscal responsibility and transparency regarding the spending of our shared resources by executive leaders in healthcare.

Motivated By Money

The general American population is unknowingly supporting executive leaders becoming very rich off of the sick and our limited healthcare dollars. I am forced to come to only one conclusion: they want to keep us sick.

"They" being those who have the power and authority in healthcare, those that have the ability to shape and control the status quo, incumbents, those that support the current system, and the ones who are getting extremely wealthy at the expense of our health.

The tactics and processes used and decisions made by these leaders in healthcare are all for the promotion of keeping us sick, so we will continue to utilize the system and contribute to their bottom-lines. This is why our system is in the current dysfunctional state that it is in.

They want to keep us sick because they are making a great deal of money from it.

American Writer Rusty Eric once warned us that... $\longrightarrow$

"As long as *greed* **is** *stronger* **than compassion, there will always be** *suffering.***"**
-Rusty Eric

So, what does one do when they have arrived at this place?

I have to say that it was a *sad* day for me when I came to this realization as a researcher, writer, and professor.

- -

1. Then, immediately, I realized that there were only three things I could do next: stay healthy, be an informed healthcare consumer, and be an advocate for others.

It wasn't my first hypothesis; although, I knew that our system needed *help*.

I just wasn't sure exactly what kind or why.

2. I know these words are bold statements, but my philosophy is that bold facts must be met with bold responses.

Part 3

How You You Should- About It ⟶

Can **-And**
Do Something!

Before starting, please take five minutes to reflect upon the quote on the following page. Feel free to use the space provided below to write, draw or sketch anything that comes to your mind.

"Revolution is not a one time event."
— Audre Lorde

Chapter 7

Stay
Healthy

If they want me *sick*, the first thing I can to do is stay healthy.

That was my initial thought after digesting this data.

It became my goal to stay healthy, so I would have no reason to utilize the system except for preventative services. Unfortunately and unsurprisingly, the U.S. healthcare system doesn't prioritize prevention as it should.

In my opinion, emphasis should be moved from treatment to prevention—from sick care to health care as one of many solutions to the current healthcare crisis.

Prevention means deterring the development of disease before symptoms or life-threatening events occur.

A focus on prevention does not imply that disease can be eliminated but rather reduces its incidence, acuteness, and severity—and subsequently, its use of healthcare system resources.

The old metaphor stated by Benjamin Franklin is true:

"An ounce of prevention is worth a pound of cure."

A 2017 systematic review of the return on investment of public health interventions in high-income countries found a median return of 14 to 1.

Confirming that prevention does, in fact, <u>save</u> money.

Did You ? Know?

Public health interventions and prevention opportunities such as childhood vaccinations, mammograms, school-based violence prevention programs, indoor smoking bans, healthy food retailers in low-income neighborhoods, and other prevention activities improve health outcomes and prevent illness and death.

Stay Healthy

In 1850, politician Lemuel Shattuck surveyed the state of Massachusetts to make recommendations for the promotion of public and personal health and wrote the Report of the Sanitary Commission of Massachusetts. He found that death and disease could be prevented; prevention could save more lives than cure, and prevention can limit the drain of limited resources.

Many civic and local infrastructure changes were made in response to this report, such as building a sewage system and proper refuse disposal, and since then, this has been found to be attributed to a 30 year increase in our life expectancy.

Efforts to expand prevention continue to be obstructed by a system better suited for profit from acute and specialty care. As a result, prevention and public health are continually marginalized.

As noted previously, economic incentives encourage overuse of services by favoring procedural over intellectual tasks, such as surgery instead of behavior-change advising and specialty over primary care.

Medical school education must be updated to address psychological, social and economic determinants of disease and not just generalized disease diagnosis and treatment approaches. This is because it has long been recognized and determined by research that our behaviors, framed by our physical and social environments, are the primary determinants of our health and well-being.

Furthermore, insurance companies and other payers will need to reimburse for health maintenance and prevention activities instead of disease identification and treatment. This requires a nondiscriminatory system that ensures everyone has access to affordable health coverage, so prevention opportunities are utilized and not addressed in the emergency room when an acute situation occurs as a result of being uninsured.

Hippocrates, a Greek physician known as the father of Western medicine, noted more than 2000 years ago that

"it's far more important to know what person the disease has than what disease the person has."

All of this requires *re-emphasis* on the importance of *primary* care versus *specialty* care; prevention occurs within the primary care environment.

Studies confirm that reinvigorating primary care can improve quality and reduce costs. According to the Dartmouth Institute for Health Policy and Clinical Practice, the U.S. states that rely more on primary care have lower Medicare spending, lower resource usage (hospital beds, physician labor), lower utilization rates (physician visits, days in the ICU), and better quality of care (fewer ICU deaths and a higher composite quality score). An imbalance between primary and specialty care has been an issue for decades. An analysis published in Health Affairs noted that from 2005 to 2015, the number of primary care physicians increased by only 8%, and the number of specialists increased 48%.

Further, the Association of American Medical Colleges noted in a report that the proportion of practicing physicians in 2016 in the U.S. was 68% specialists and 32% primary care physicians.

This directly reduces prevention and case management opportunities and replaces those with a high volume of intensive, expensive, and invasive procedures.

The motivation, again, may be money over service; choosing specialty over primary care often means a larger paycheck.

Family Medicine, Pediatrics, and Public Health and Preventative Medicine are consistently among the lowest paid in Medscape's annual physician compensation report.

What is even more compelling is that some of the higher-earning specialties, such as orthopedics and plastic surgery, report lower levels of satisfaction with their compensation, even though they are close to making double of what primary care physicians make.

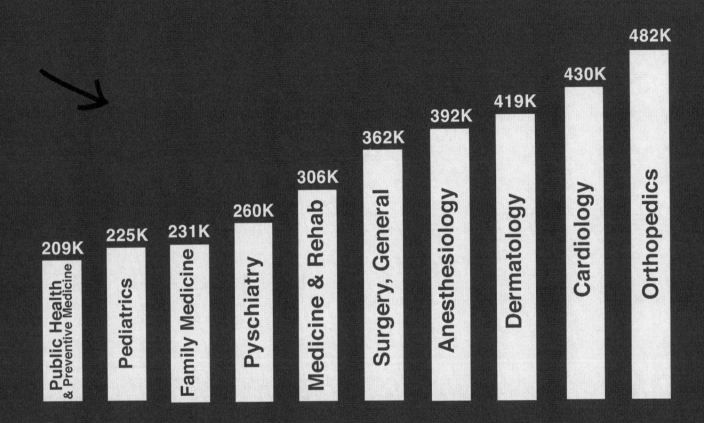

Annual Average Physician Compensation

Based on Specialty

Source: Medscape Physician Compensation Report 2019

Even *more* paradoxical is that the nation's public health system...

is responsible for preventing disease and improving the health of Americans but has been consistently underfunded for decades.

In 2017, public health represented just 3% of all federal health spending in the U.S., and all states regularly report budget cuts in their public health programs. In 2018, 17 states cut their public health funding.

Although we only spend a small percentage of our federal and state budgets on prevention and other public health initiatives, it has been found to impact people and communities tremendously.

Imagine the impact on communities and people if we budgeted more.

CDC's State Physical Activity and Nutrition (SPAN) Program

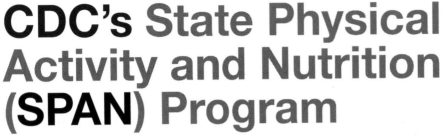

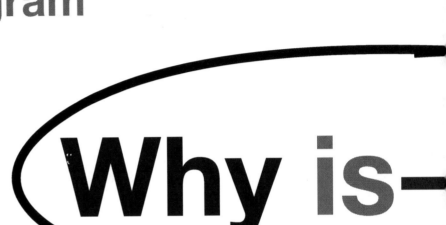

Why is—

Which focuses on **improving** nutrition and **encouraging** physical activity through...

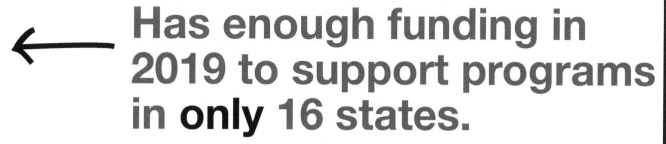

Has enough funding in 2019 to support programs in **only** 16 states.

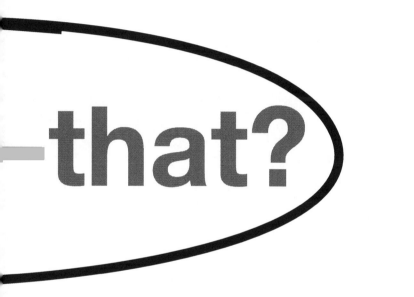

—that?

Education, breastfeeding, nutrition guidelines, street design, and other **local efforts**

Stay Healthy

I have been a governor-appointed Public Health Official on a state of Illinois public health board since 2015 with many other incredibly dedicated public health advocates.

We get together and develop plans for all of the ways we could improve the health of Illinois residents, but never are we able to obtain funding to implement any of them. We dreamed up plans for tackling mental health issues, chronic diseases, and promoted ways to encourage healthy eating, but dreams they stayed.

However, they were documented, nonetheless, in case funding should ever come through. For the year 2019, the state of Illinois only provided 1% of overall state appropriations to the Illinois Department of Public Health, leaving yet another year for our plans to collect dust on the internet.

Most states have a similar story.

Our only hope is for lawmakers to prioritize and invest more in prevention and public health.

One move towards this goal was the development of the Prevention and Public Health Fund, established by the ACA as the first dedicated and mandatory funding source for prevention and public health within the federal budget.

The goal of this tax-payer fund is to expand and sustain national investments in evidence-based strategies in prevention and public health programs. The Prevention Fund will provide $14.5 billion over 10 years (2015-2025). However, this fund has been repeatedly cut and used to pay for other legislation.

For example, the fund will lose $1.35 billion over 10 years under the Bipartisan Budget Act of 2018, implemented by the Trump administration.

A Real Life

Life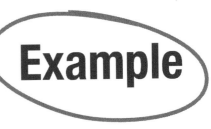

The YMCA's Diabetes Prevention Program is an example of an evidence-based strategy supported by the Prevention and Public Health Fund. YMCA-trained lifestyle coaches administer a one-year, group-based intervention promoting healthy eating and physical activity for people with pre-diabetes. Program results found participants lost 5% to 7% of their body weight, significantly reducing their likelihood of developing type-2 diabetes. This data incentivized more than 60 health insurance plans to cover the cost of the Diabetes Prevention Program *because the costs of the program were far less than the cost of covering a diabetic patient.*

Stay Healthy

How does one stay healthy when we live in an environment where prevention and maintaining health is not culturally or politically prioritized, and leaders are kept very wealthy by keeping us sick? It took me several years to figure this out; especially because health is relative and defined differently by everyone.

This is what the trendy "patient-centered" care concept is all about.

For me, this is massages, yoga, vacation, and vitamin D supplements. For my husband, it's cycling, the chiropractor, and Netflix documentaries. For my daughter, it's meditation, reading, and healthy eating, and for my good friend, it's dancing, therapy, and red wine. We are all challenged to figure out what healthy means for us. For one person, this might mean eating one less fast food meal a week, going to one's yearly physical for routine blood work, reducing one's sugar intake, going to the gym one more day a week, or eating more veggies.

We are all unique with different internal body chemistry requirements, past experiences, and health needs.

We all ultimately know what we need and what's best for us. It just takes time to reflect on it, experiment, and figure it out. So many of us have been taught to leave it to our doctor to figure it out for us, and that needs to end. We need to become active participants in our health and take back power and control of our own well-being.

Of course, this is going to take some effort. It took me several years, one step at a time, to figure out what it was that I needed for my wellness, but I made it a priority, which is key. I have spent hours upon hours researching to help me understand how to feel better. I have experimented and found what works for me.

I recommend working with your intuition and a primary care doctor, functional medicine practitioner, or local naturopathic doctor to help you discover what this means for you.

On the following pages I display what I have learned about my own health needs and what keeps me healthy and out of the healthcare system. May this just be a general guide for you as you begin your own path to personal health and wellbeing.

→ 1. Eating Differently

It started by giving up soda, then refined and added sugars (which happen to be in just about everything.) This alone did wonders for my energy, mood, and body weight. Then, I began to eat more plant forward, meaning, more fruits, veggies, legumes, and leafy greens in exchange for less meat, dairy, and eggs. Some personal aliments I had been struggling with had disappeared (sinus issues, headaches, acne).

Next, I began to purchase more organic products to reduce my exposure to pesticides, and eventually, I ended up having four garden beds in my backyard and a compost bin to grow my own organics. I began to notice how differently home-grown and unprocessed food tasted, and my body began to crave it. Sure, I began to spend more time in the kitchen making my own meals, batches of bread and marinara from scratch, but the time investment has contributed tremendously to the bottom line of my health.

→ 2. Exercising Regularly

I have always been an active person throughout my life. The need for movement comes naturally for me. It started off as ballet and karate as a child, then dance and yoga when I got into my twenties. As I got older, this changed to running and cycling, and now, I train year-round to do duathlons and triathlons. The beauty of exercise is that it comes in so many different forms: basketball, tennis, swimming, walking, Tai Chi, and so much more. The key is finding what you enjoy, and that is different for everyone.

I eventually understood that the main purpose for exercising is to keep my heart and other important muscles strong, and burning calories is just a small part of it. I had terrible, achy knee joints, and it wasn't until I started running that I built strength and muscle around my knees to support my body's needs better, and the achiness went away. I also realized that in order for this to be sustainable, it must be a lifestyle change. Simply working out for a few months and then stopping will not work. Making exercise, in whatever form, a regular part of your life is key.

→ 3. Reduce Chemical Exposure

Chemicals we use every day are altering what's primal to us, leading cancer to become more prevalent. Parts of our genome simply cannot survive a situation where the environment suffers from the full overload of toxins we currently live with. Through cancer and disease, our bodies are working out new genomic defects and experimenting to see what survives. Unfortunately, we cannot evolve as fast as what we are exposing ourselves to via the chemicals in the foods we eat, the air we breathe, and the products we use.

Once I realized this, I began to slowly reduce my exposure to chemicals, and the process was eye-opening as I discovered how much we are exposed to: produce, dish soap, shampoo, dryer sheets, lotion, makeup, cleaning supplies, feminine products, and so much more. One at a time, I began to change what I purchased and began to rely more on natural products. Sure, this increases my spending, but again, I look at it as an investment in my health, and soon enough, as demand increases, prices will reduce.

→ **4. Meditation**

Nothing has impacted my life more than meditation. I started by doing a 30-day challenge, meditating every day for 30 days straight, and it changed my life more than I ever expected it to. It started at a time when life was a bit much for me to handle, and now it is forever embedded as a part of my daily life. Most people are not aware of the impact modern living has on ourselves; all around us is an epidemic of poor emotional, physical, psychological, philosophical, behavioral, social, and spiritual health. Everyone is dealing with too much. These are the side effects of negativity, fear, inequality, capitalism, and patriarchy.

I, too, was stuck right in it. The amazing thing is that I realized that I get to decide how I want to feel. When we are out of alignment with our inner light and spiritual space, there are physical implications. Meditation helped me reconnect with my inner power, which helped me to have better relationships, mental health, responses to stress, self-awareness, less anxiety, and helped me rid addiction from my life. Modern society wants us to go, go, go, but in reality, what we need for proper functioning is rest and silence. This is because we are not just physical beings; we are also spiritual beings. By connecting to our inner light and taking the time with ourselves to process emotions, we will ultimately become healthier overall with a sense of well-being and gratitude. Greek philosopher Plato once said, "You ought not to attempt to cure the eyes without the head or the head without the body, so neither ought you attempt to cure the body without the soul… for the part can never be well unless the whole is well."

→ 5. Supplement as necessary

It is an unfortunate reality that our modern lifestyle has created a situation where our bodies are missing key nutrients due to the soil our food is grown in, how our food is cooked, how often we exercise, get sunlight, sleep, and relax. Modern living has our internal body chemistry out of balance and as a result, requires us to supplement. B-12, iron, multivitamins, and fiber are just a few typical supplements used by many. A few that I use are primarily to help boost my immune system. We all must befriend germs. We live symbiotically with them. Allowing our immune system to interact with them is necessary, so we can build up immunities for a healthy future response. In order to befriend germs, we must fix our gut (that is our intestinal tract.)

A lot of recent research has revealed the connection between our gut health and immune health. Because our processed, American diet wreaks havoc on our gut, we must repair it. It is estimated that most of the American population has what is called a leaky gut (also called intestinal permeability), leading to allergies, autoimmune diseases, pain, inflammation, and more. Hippocrates suggested long ago that all disease begins in the gut, and he was right. Probiotics and L-glutamine supplements have been found to fix these leaks in our gut and allow for healthy bacteria to live there, which allows our immune system to function more effectively. Vitamin D also assists in this process, and since taking these three supplements, I have been able to manage my diverticulosis without surgery, have eliminated irritable bowel syndrome that I struggled with for years, and reduced my need for antibiotics when I am fighting a cold or virus.

Chapter 8

Be Informed

We <u>know</u> *so much* about what's going on with Kanye West, Donald Trump's *latest* Tweet...

the show we recently finished binge watching, and the spreadsheet at work you spent weeks mastering. We spend time researching the hotels we want to stay at while on vacation or the best schools to send our children to, but most of us aren't as informed about our own personal health and healthcare rights. This is on purpose. Why would they want us to know that they want to keep us sick when they can make money from it? The last thing these healthcare leaders want is the power that comes from an informed consumer market. Those who want us sick are banking on the ignorance of society.

Consumers are kept out of the loop on purpose to preserve the status quo and by being fed distracting lies through the media that we constantly consume.

This is why I prefaced this book by noting that 90% of us are unaware of the information presented here. Imagine the power health consumers could have if 90% of us knew the information in this book. Becoming an informed healthcare consumer begins with the relationships we have with our doctors.

The physician-patient relationship is foundational to healthcare. It is the bedrock of our system and is based on trust. This relationship begins when treatment is rendered and ends when treatment is no longer needed. Once created, the relationship imposes legal obligations for the physician to provide medical care that falls within a standard of care: obtain consent, maintain confidentiality, and provide continuity of care.

Providing informed consent is the first step healthcare consumers can take to become informed and active participants in their healthcare.

Fully informed consent is a critical element of good medical care. The way a doctor communicates with their patient is important, especially when discussing the pros and cons of treatment.

Be Informed

The American Medical Association states that the process of informed consent occurs when communication between a patient and physician results in the patient's agreement to undergo a specific medical intervention.

Patients have the right to receive information and ask questions about recommended treatments, so they can make well-considered decisions about care.

The word "informed" in the term "informed consent" means having knowledge or understanding of the facts.

- -

We are in the *driver seat* of our health when we are *informed* healthcare consumers.

Moral issues are at the basis of laws regarding informed consent. In 1962, 8,000 babies were born deformed due to their mothers having taken a sleeping-pill-tranquilizer called "thalidomide" (a drug not approved by the FDA for use in pregnant women due to a lack of substantial evidence of safety).

After this tragedy, a Federal Consumer Bill of Rights was proclaimed: the right to safety, the right to be informed, the right to choose, and the right to be heard. Informed consent is more than just a document that needs to be signed; it is an ethical and legal obligation of physician duty. Informed consent is an on-going dialogue between a patient and their doctor.

Throughout the U.S. there are different rules and regulations in each state regarding consent; there isn't any Federal protection.

The general rule, typical to most state laws, is that informed consent must be obtained by a doctor prior to treatment of any kind, and consent may be oral, written, or even implied.

Did You — Know?

?

Even though some form of informed consent laws have been in place since the Consumer Bill of Rights in the 60s, things like this still unfortunately happen: A bill to ban sterilization surgeries on inmates in California prisons days after an audit showed officials failed to follow the state's rules for obtaining consent for the procedures. The bill unanimously passed the assembly health committee as lawmakers scrambled to respond to the audit, which showed that errors were made in obtaining informed consent from 39 women inmates who had their fallopian tubes tied while incarcerated between 2005 and 2011.

Source: Reuters 2014 - Ban On Inmate Sterilizations Moves Forward In California Legislature

Be Informed

Respecting a person's right to determine what happens to their own body and full disclosure of risks involved prior to treatment is an expression of the ethical principle of autonomy. Patients have the right to make their own decisions, choose the type of treatment, and refuse the treatment altogether.

This act of self-determination also includes who will do the treatment, when, and where. Americans value autonomy, and it is impossible to achieve within a physician-patient relationship unless a proper informed consent process has been implemented.

Many physicians are *very* <u>nonchalant</u> about informed consent, and I have observed *one too many* doctors not do a thorough job.

Generally, state laws point out that disclosure to patients must include: the patient's condition, nature of proposed treatment, benefits expected from treatment and potential risks, treatment alternatives with their benefits and risks, and the name of the healthcare provider who is to perform the procedure.

Physicians should avoid technical terms, answer questions, request if understanding was obtained, and invite questions. All of this information should help competent individuals make informed decisions about their healthcare. The term "competent" is important here because only patients with the mental capacity to make informed decisions about medical care retain that right. If because of age, intoxication, injury, illness, emotional stress, mental disability, or other reasons, a healthcare provider can decide that a patient does not have decision-making capacity and may not be able to exercise autonomy.

This is very critical in end-of-life decision making because many individuals at the end of their life are incapacitated in one way or another, no matter what the age.

A Real Life

Life #1

Submit your healthcare story at toerrishealthcare.com/stories

"Our 1 year old son needed to have some diagnostic tests to determine the cause of his non-typical asthma symptoms. These included an endoscopy to look at his upper airway for obstructions and imaging of his brain and chest. The imaging was to be done while he was still under anesthesia, and originally, the physician requested a CT scan. At this point our son had several CT scans already, and we were concerned about another one. Upon doing research, we realized that an MRI is another option with much less radiation exposure. We brought this to the attention of our son's physician, and he told us that he originally chose CT scan over MRI because it's faster and would require our son to be under anesthesia, which has risks of its own, for less time. We were upset because the physician did not give us the option to choose what we felt was best for our son (being under anesthesia for longer with less radiation or more radiation exposure but less time spent under anesthesia) and instead made the choice for us with his original CT scan order. Our autonomy was stripped away from us, and we didn't even notice it. If it wasn't for our own gut feeling and time spent doing research, we would not have been active and informed participants in our son's care because the physician didn't give us that option."

Did You — Know?

?

To maximize surgery time, surgeons often schedule overlapping surgeries. Concurrent surgery is the term used when a doctor is simultaneously booked in two separate rooms at the same time. This is typical of busy operating rooms, preparation and procedure for one patient begins in one room as the care of another patient finishes in another room. As of 2016, surgeons are required to inform a patient if a surgeon will be performing overlapping surgery due to updated guidelines from the American College of Surgeons. This was following several lawsuits that surfaced regarding complications resulting among patients whose surgeons were performing overlapping surgery. These are only guidelines and not backed by legislative regulation. Instead, only guidance was provided by the U.S. Senate in 2016 stating that a well-designed informed consent policy should include a discussion of a surgeon's possible absence during part of the patient's surgery. As a result, most lawsuits will reside with the physician as no law states this as a requirement and is normally done in the daily operating room.

Be Informed

We plan everything—our schedules, our careers and work projects, our weddings and vacations, our retirements—but rarely the end of our life.

Patients have the right to be involved in end-of-life decisions and may exercise their autonomy by executing different types of advance directives. These are instructions that outline one's desires regarding medical care, should they become unable to make these decisions.

This includes usage of life-sustaining treatment, such as artificial feeding, mechanical ventilators, resuscitation, defibrillation, antibiotics, dialysis, and other invasive procedures. If we don't exercise this right, then other people will make those decisions for us.

These people could be our family members or, if unavailable, the physicians themselves. Ideally, we want to make our own decisions, not somebody else who may have different morals, values, or beliefs than we do.

Advance directive laws vary from state to state and are considered legal documents that must be signed.

Another very effective and immediate way of being more engaged and informed regarding one's healthcare is by having copies of one's medical records.

These can help individuals become better informed about their medical history and more engaged in their own healthcare. In fact, 8 in 10 individuals who have viewed their medical records online considered the information useful. Reviewing your medical records is not only a smart thing to do, it's your right. I have to admit that it was an eye-opening experience for me when I requested medical records for myself and my kids. I had found errors and additional information I was never given.

Reviewing commentary by nurses and doctors is also an eye-opening experience. The Federal Health Insurance Portability and Accountability Act (HIPAA) guarantees all patients a copy of their medical records within 30 days of requesting them. There is usually a small cost to this, because providers can reasonably charge for copying and mailing the records, but this small cost is worth the outcome of being more informed.

A Real Life

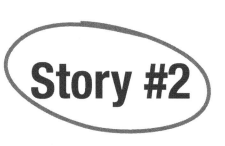

Story #2

Submit your healthcare story at toerrishealthcare.com/stories

"I had a chest X-ray done during the flu season when I visited my local emergency room when I was very sick and had trouble breathing. The results didn't show anything worrisome. I just needed time to rest and inhalers to help me breathe as the upper respiratory virus worked through its lifecycle. I was inspired to order my medical records from that visit after a friend recently did the same and found the records to be beneficial to her. When I received the records the chest x-ray showed that I had mild levoscoliosis (curvature of the spine). I would have never known if I didn't order my records because none of my doctors mentioned this was noticed by the radiologist on my imaging. Why didn't anyone find it important to mention this to me? Levoscoliosis can be a serious condition and explains some of the other symptoms I had been dealing with."

One of the *main reasons* for market failure in the healthcare industry is because we are *uninformed* consumers.

Neil Postman, American author, educator, and media theorist, wrote in 1985 that

> *"Americans are the best entertained and quite likely the least well-informed people in the Western world."*

Several surveys confirm this. McKinsey found that many consumers misunderstand the sources of healthcare costs.

A Kaiser Health Tracking Poll found that when asked what Americans knew about their governor's decision on whether to expand Medicaid in their state, 78% said they hadn't heard enough to say whether the governor had announced a decision or what that decision was.

It also found that gaps in knowledge persisted three years after the passage of the ACA; a majority of Americans, 57%, say they do not have enough information about the law to understand how it will affect them.

At the same time, many Americans hold misimpressions about the law.

57% mistakenly think the law creates a government-run health plan (the so-called "public option"). A National Public Radio (NPR) survey found that 43% "don't know" if passage of the ACA caused Medicare spending to decrease.

The University of Chicago found that over half of Americans say they received a medical bill they thought was covered by insurance or where the amount they owed was higher than expected.

Because healthcare is considered to be a commodity in the U.S., there are factors affecting the price, demand, and availability of it. The market forces prices up when supply declines and demand rises and drives them down when supply grows or demand contracts.

Be Informed

Healthcare is not insulated from conventional market forces that operate in the rest of the economy. Economists know that in an ideal market it is assumed that there are a large number of sellers, so no one can greatly determine the price. It's also assumed that both buyers and sellers are well informed and aware of changes in prices, and goods and services bought and sold are homogeneous, so buyers make decisions primarily on price.

Further, some of the standard market forces that affect supply and demand include weather, cost of gasoline, elections, terrorism, downturns in the economy, changes in the stock market, availability of materials, and technological advancement.

But economists also know that these standard market forces aren't always applied in the same way in the healthcare industry because patients are uninformed about hospital quality and insurance, reducing incentives to shop for better deals. Therefore, poorly performing hospitals do not feel demand-side pressure from patients to improve quality, so a poor correlation between hospital performance and market share exists.

Because pricing transparency doesn't exist, providers and insurers drive utilization, not patients. Other forces that keep the healthcare industry unable to function as an ideal market include: information not being easily available or understandable, consolidation in the industry reduces choice and increases monopolies, and lobbying by the pharmaceutical industry controls prices.

Those who are proponents of market-based reform must know that there is an inherent problem in the simple market economy philosophy of eliminating waste and escalating costs by strengthening competition. Healthcare is not like any other market in the economy because the consumers do not directly pay for the service or know the cost. Our choices are limited and many are chosen for us. Additionally, public health advocates, like myself, argue that it's also a human right, unlike the other commodities purchased on the open market. Therefore, government intervention is required. Our current fragmented system that is in shambles is a result of healthcare functioning as a market-based commodity product.

Why would we think the status quo will continue to work?

To *save* our healthcare system, we must *gain power* as consumers.

When healthcare consumers are informed and engaged, it challenges decision-makers to consider consumer-driven options for healthcare delivery. In order to achieve this, the system must begin with making transparency a priority. When health organizations are transparent, consumers are able to make better decisions about their purchases and utilization. Simplified, transparency means easy to see. The push to bring transparency to healthcare pricing and quality has been going on for years, but still, the industry remains one of the nation's most hazy. We must no longer remain consumers in the dark if we want transformation of our healthcare system to occur.

The pressure is on for insurers, providers, and drugmakers to offer price and quality data due to legislation written into the ACA as patient protections. A handful of these include the following: $\longrightarrow$

Hospitals are required to make their prices transparent by publishing their list prices for all of the services they provide. Hospitals must publish this information on their website in a printer or computer-friendly format.

 Insurance companies are now required to disclose rate increases of 10% or more and justify these increases to their customers, and the Department of Health and Human Services and the states have the authority to determine whether these increases are reasonable. You can find all of this information about rate increases in your state at: www.companyprofiles.healthcare.gov

---

 Insurance companies are now required to reveal the amount of your premium dollars that are actually spent on healthcare benefits and improving quality versus how much they spend on administration, such as salaries, bonuses, and marketing. If your insurance company spends less than 80% of premiums on healthcare benefits and quality, they must provide a rebate of the portion of premium dollars that exceeded this limit. Your insurance company will send you a letter every year to tell you if they missed the 80/20 mark and, therefore, owe you a rebate on your premium payments.

 Health insurance plans are required to disclose the following information and make it publicly available: claims payment policies and practices, data on the number of claims that are denied, and data on rating practices.

Be Informed

Additional legislation that has been around since 2006 has been putting pressure on hospitals to publicly display the results of their report cards, customer service scores, and ratings for measures in which they are evaluated by the various governmental agencies administering them. Some of these measures are even more important now because they are tied to financial incentives and reimbursements.

The HCAHPS (Hospital Consumer Assessment of Healthcare Providers and Systems) survey is the first national, standardized, publicly reported survey of patients' perspectives on hospital care. This survey produces data about patients' perspectives on care and links this quality data to payment.

Why?

Because data from these results creates new incentives for hospitals to improve quality of care, enhances accountability by increasing transparency to patients, and paves the way for a new, performance-based reimbursement system instead of the traditional Fee-For-Service (FFS) system.

Eleven HCAHPS measures are publicly reported on the Hospital Compare website, www.medicare.gov/hospitalcompare. Data from this survey and several others has formed the basis for report cards and other tools to help consumers understand and compare options within healthcare.

This means that the public has much more power than it has ever had before. They just don't know it yet. Most patients aren't aware that this data exists. Hospitals and insurance companies are not making it known that this information exists. They are not proudly displaying their quality report cards.

Now that you *know*, check out some of these tools on the next *page* and gain more consumer power.

→ The ACA requires healthcare providers to report recipients of gifts or payments, under the Physician Sunshine Act, by drug and medical device companies. Open Payments is a national disclosure program that makes the financial relationships between manufacturers, group purchasing organizations, and healthcare providers available to the public.
www.openpaymentsdata.cms.gov

→ Look up your hospital to see if it is being penalized by Medicare. The ACA allows the Federal government to cut payments to hospitals that have high rates of readmissions and those with the highest numbers of infections and patient injuries.
www.khn.org/news/hospital-penalties

→ The Advisory Board publishes a map that displays final pay-for-performance payment adjustments for the selected year. These are adjustments due to penalties for sub-par quality based on pay-for-performance programs.
www.sca.advisory.com/Maps/?var=p4p

→ Physician Compare is designed to help consumers make informed choices about the healthcare they receive through Medicare by comparing quality scores of different providers.
www.medicare.gov/physiciancompare

→ Find out how safe your hospital is. Leapfrog Group provides a safety grade that is the gold standard measure of patient safety that includes data on errors, injuries, accidents, and infections.
www.hospitalsafetyscore.org

→ ProPublica calculated death and complication rates for surgeons performing one of eight elective procedures in Medicare, so patients can use their database to know more about a surgeon before their operation.
www.projects.propublica.org/surgeons

- -

As this era of transparency in healthcare continues to evolve and entrepreneurs
Start to become familiar with some of these that are currently available,
Make a pledge to be an informed healthcare consumer by making conscious

→ Healthgrades is the leader in making information on physicians and hospitals more accessible and transparent. Consumers can search patient satisfaction and quality scores, review experiences with doctors, and read others' reviews as well.
www.healthgrades.com
www.healthgrades.com/quality/ratings-awards/reports

→ The American Federation of Labor and Congress of Industrial Organizations (AFL-CIO) maintains a public list, called Paywatch, of the highest paid CEO's in each industry sector. Select the healthcare industry and your specific state to narrow down the results, and learn more about the imbalance in our economy between the pay of CEO's and working people in your state.
www.aflcio.org/paywatch/highest-paid-ceos

→ Every state has some sort of health report card for its citizens. Look up your state in the IPRO state report card directory.
www.abouthealthtransparency.org/report-card-directory

→ This site highlights journalists working to bring transparency to the system by informing patients of the prices of health procedures and supplies.
www.clearhealthcosts.com

→ You can easily search any procedure to find out how much you should be paying in your area with Healthcare Blue Book.
www.healthcarebluebook.com

☆ **Stay *Healthy*, Be *Informed*!** ☆

- -

→ **take advantage of this large opportunity, new online tools will be developed.**
→ **and don't just live on autopilot—question, research, and be informed.**
→ **and educated choices in your decision-making.**

Chapter 9

Be
An
Advocate

Our United States healthcare system is *dysfunctional*.

It leaves many without coverage, is the most expensive in the world, and drives many into bankruptcy and poor health outcomes. Our two-tiered system of care maintains access for Americans with comfortable incomes but restricts access for everyone else, noted by Anthony Kovner, PhD, as a particularly brutal form of rationing.

The majority of us agree that things must change, but we hardly make much progress because we can't seem to find something that unites us all in our great healthcare debate. I contend that there actually is common ground. President Donald Trump once noted,

"Nobody knew healthcare could be so complicated."

However, at its core, it really isn't.

Universal Health Coverage is one of the most widely shared goals in public health around the globe. While countries debate (and then implement) different funding mechanisms, they focus less on how healthcare is funded and, instead, more on who has access.

There are two specific instances where the United Nations (U.N.) unanimously declared Universal Health Coverage as a public priority for our world.

As noted in part one, the first was in 1948 when 48 member countries signed the Universal Declaration of Human Rights, agreeing that all member countries would ensure their citizens have the right to adequate healthcare as a public good and not a commodity.

Then again, more recently, with the Sustainable Development Goals of 2015 stating that all U.N. member states agree to try and achieve Universal Health Coverage by 2030, urging governments to move toward providing all people with access to affordable, quality healthcare services as a part of sustaining our human race and planet.

Be An Advocate

Only the developed, industrialized countries—thirty to forty of the world's two-hundred countries—have established healthcare systems.

Each country devises its own set of arrangements for meeting the three basic goals of a healthcare system: keeping people healthy, treating the sick, and protecting families against financial ruin from medical bills.

Developed countries around the world have achieved Universal Health Coverage in several ways. None of them trust the free market completely and, instead, impose regulations like insurance companies accepting everyone and not making a profit on basic care.

Everyone is mandated to buy insurance, often shared by employer and employee contributions, while the government pays premiums for the poor, and doctors and hospitals have to accept a standard set of fixed prices.

Additionally, not all of the countries do what's considered socialized medicine; instead, many have private doctors and hospitals as a part of the equation.

Let me *repeat* that— single-payer healthcare *does not* automatically mean socialized medicine.

The biggest challenges our country has right now are how to best structure health coverage to maximize health and value and how much public spending we want to devote to subsidizing coverage for people who cannot afford it.

The World Health Organization had its 1st Global Symposium on Health System Research in 2010 and concluded with this summary: Out of the countries in their analysis, 75 had legislation that provided a mandate for Universal Health Coverage independent of income.

The U.S. was still not one of them.

Be An Advocate

I reached out to a woman who works for the World Health Organization to get some information regarding accountability toward these goals. I was told that the Universal Health Coverage goals are all aspirational, and no member country is obligated to anything other than their citizens. There will be no sanctions or the like on the U.S. for not adhering to these goals. We, as American citizens, have to take it up with our government for not doing so. The United Nations will not. It all begins with the idea that healthcare is a right. This comes naturally for me, and I share this sentiment with the majority of the population, as well. Gallup, The Journal and Pew Research polls show that most people believe it's the job of the government to ensure healthcare as a right to their citizens.

In other countries, healthcare is treated like any other public service, similar to how public libraries and police forces are financed by the government and controlled through progressive citizen tax money. Imagine if you had to give a credit card number before the police come to your 9-1-1 call. Our right to healthcare is in parallel with the right to public safety or even public library access. Keeping people safe with a police force benefits entire communities. The same goes for keeping people healthy.

It affects their entire communities: work, home, and neighborhood. This public service philosophy is noticeably universal in every other part of the developed world. Healthcare is viewed in the same way as being able to use public roads for driving.

When I speak to people about whether or not healthcare is a right, some say "no" and that it should be paid for on one's own. With a single-payer healthcare system, everyone pays their fair share when their taxes are filed. Many of the people who are currently not paying would be. Simply framed, single-payer means that we pay taxes to the government based on how much we make, and in return, we are provided a universal healthcare plan with necessary basics that everyone is entitled to. The government then becomes the single-payer in our healthcare. The same applies for how public education is provided. We pay taxes. They plan and manage the system, and we show up to school. Our role, other than paying taxes, is to elect people who can rally for our education needs and hope our interests get a say in policy.

We are the only industrialized country in the world that does not treat healthcare in this fashion.

The right to healthcare *actually* saves lives and money.

Studies show that lack of health insurance is associated with an increased risk of death among the uninsured. Expanding coverage to all will save the system money because the uninsured are not only an ethical problem but also, a fiscal concern. Coverage expansions significantly increase patients' health and wellbeing because access to primary care can lower overall healthcare utilization. Increasing access to preventive services will subsequently lower disease rates, which cost the system a significant amount of money. Other benefits manifest as better medication adherence, better management of chronic conditions, reduced reliance on emergency care, and psychological well-being born of knowing one has coverage when getting sick or hurt.

When people have access to healthcare, they live healthier lives and miss work less, allowing them to contribute more to the economy.

Norman Daniels, PhD, an ethics professor at Harvard University, put it this way, "Healthcare preserves for people the ability to participate in the political, social, and economic life of society. It sustains them as fully participating citizens." In the U.S., we are 33% less likely to have a regular doctor, 25% more likely to have unmet health needs, and over 50% more likely to not obtain needed medications compared to our Canadian counterparts who have a universal right to healthcare through single-payer coverage.

Consider what happens when one cannot get their medications when they have a chronic disease, such as high blood pressure or Parkinson's. One could end up in the emergency room, increase disease progression further and create a lower quality of life, strain relationships because they are depressed, lose their job because they can't effectively work, or end up with an addiction to help ease their pains.

This type of life costs more than the one that has access to health coverage and sees their primary care doctor regularly for medication and wellness checks. Economic studies have shown that this is true.

One study published by the Journal of the American Medical Association found that preventable causes of death are estimated to be responsible for 900,000 deaths annually, which translates to nearly 40% of the total yearly mortality in the United States. The Surgeon General estimates that increasing the use of preventative services to the recommended levels could save $3.7 billion in medical costs annually.

Not only does giving people access to health coverage *save* the system money, it also allows for people to live a *better* quality of life. Don't we *want* that for our fellow human beings?

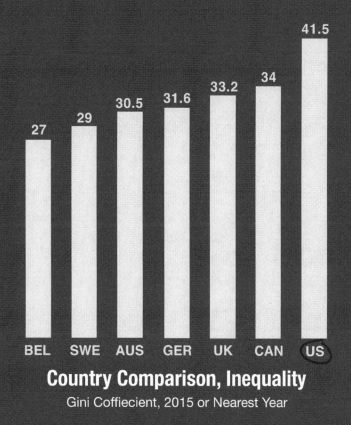

Country Comparison, Inequality
Gini Coffiecient, 2015 or Nearest Year

Source: Peterson-Kaiser Health System Tracker

Being poor is perhaps the single largest determinant of health status. A large body of research has demonstrated the many ways in which income can influence health outcomes. People with lower incomes are less likely than those with higher incomes to report being in good health, and there is a growing disparity in the life expectancies of low and high income Americans. The GINI coefficient is a measure of this income inequality, a characteristic the U.S. leads the developed world in.

Be An Advocate

Another way that universal coverage saves costs is that it will reduce uncompensated care, which is an overall measure of hospital care provided for which no payment was received from the patient or insurer.

Since 2000, hospitals of all types have provided more than $620 billion in uncompensated care to their patients. In 2017, $38 billion was spent on uncompensated care.

More importantly, providers do not bear the full impact of uncompensated care. Rather, funding is available through a wide variety of sources to help providers defray the costs associated with it.

Kaiser estimated in 2013 that $53.3 billion of taxpayer money was used to help providers offset uncompensated care costs. We are already paying for the uninsured through uncompensated care provider tax-relief. These are our public dollars.

Why don't we put that $53 billion into the system and expand coverage to keep people healthier?

There are a lot of healthcare dollars in our system; they are just used ineffectively and in the wrong places.

Beyond the examples mentioned, the Institute of Medicine estimates that we waste a half-trillion dollars annually through inefficiency. The U.S. is unlike any other country because it maintains so many separate systems for separate classes of people.

All other developed countries have settled on one model for everybody. This is much simpler than the U.S. system; it's fairer and cheaper, too.

Physicians for a National Health Program says,

> "When it comes to treating veterans, we're Britain or Cuba. For Americans over the age of 65 on Medicare, we're Canada. For working Americans who get insurance on the job, we're Germany. For the 10-15% of the population who have no health insurance, the United States is Cambodia, Burkina Faso, or rural India, with access to a doctor if you can pay the bill out-of-pocket at the time of treatment."

Be An Advocate

There are hidden costs of our system's complexity.

When managing 50 different sets of state insurance regulations for managing Medicaid, there are over 800 different health insurance companies. We all pay different premiums; every employer is a different large group, and our charges for services all differ based on provider group and insurance company. This multi-payer way of financing care directly creates an administrative burden. BMC Health Services Research estimated that moving to a single-payer healthcare system can reduce our administrative expenditures by 80%, and a simplified financing system would result in cost savings exceeding $350 billion annually. Combine all of that with the fact that we lose tens of billions of dollars to fraud a year due to this very fragmented and complex billing system. Further, the foundation for these administrative burdens stems from how we uniquely allow our healthcare system organizations to profit. We pay premiums that are inflated with insurance marketing and advertising costs, as well as multi-million-dollar compensations for executives. This is why the National Health Expenditure analysis noted that private health insurance plans spend 11.7% of premiums on administrative costs versus the 6.3% by public health programs.

Advocates of Universal Healthcare point out that the lower costs of public insurance programs (much like our own Medicare program) can provide savings on administrative spending alone that could finance much of the cost of care for the uninsured.

The U.S. Census notes that 67% of the United States get their health coverage privately (56% from employers), and 38% get public coverage financed by the government (with our tax money). This leaves 8.8% of people, or 28.5 million, who did not have health insurance at any point during the year, which is the highest rate of any developed and industrialized country in the world. Who are these people? The majority of them live in Texas and other parts of the south. They are between the ages of 19 and 64, make less than $25,000 a year, are either black or Hispanic, and live in poverty of some kind. The disparities of who has access to health coverage and who does not are very clear. The immoral nature of deep racial and ethnic disparities remains when it comes to health coverage and equity. The refusal of nearly 20 states to expand Medicaid, particularly in the south, has left hundreds of thousands of Americans with these demographics uninsured.

This **image** by the U.S. Census shows that we know how to cover the young and the old, but we have no idea what to do with the rest of the population. **You'll notice a big spike when people hit their mid-20s.** People in that age range are also less likely to have a job that offers insurance, and they're less likely to be able to afford it on their own. Many of whom are also newly **overloaded with student loan debt.**

A Kaiser survey of uninsured Americans found that 45% say that their reason for being uninsured is that **the cost is too high;** others say they lost their job or changed employers, or their **employer doesn't offer coverage at all.** If you do not get insurance through work, do not qualify for Medicaid, and you do not qualify for tax credits through the state exchanges/marketplaces (thanks to the ACA), **then healthcare is too expensive, and therefore, you go without.**

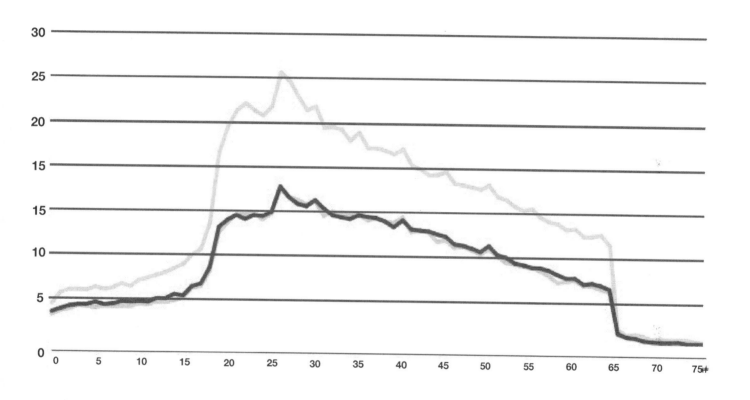

Uninsured Rate by Single Year of Age: 2013, 2016 and 2017

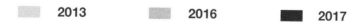

2013   2016   2017

Source: U.S Census Bureau 2013, 2016, and 2017 American Community Surveys

→ Since most people get their insurance through their employer, I believe it's important to understand the history of how and why employers got involved in healthcare as an employee benefit.

→ In the late 1920s, several hospitals in Texas joined up and formed an insurance plan called Blue Cross to help people purchase hospital services. This caught the eye of a public school system in the 1930s who realized that they needed to keep their employees healthy, so their business could run effectively. In response, they made a business deal with this local hospital insurance group to provide services to their employees.

→ This was a competitive advantage for this school system because their employees (teachers) stayed productive, leading directly to their quality and output. Other companies saw this happening and wanted in on this strategy of investing in their employees health. Unfortunately, because of the Depression, Congress was forced to pass the Stabilization Act of 1942, which instituted wage freezes for all the nation's workers. Businesses began to wonder how they would retain workers if they couldn't give raises. Insurance companies pressed their case through marketing campaigns, and the allure of fringe benefits became front and center. Then in 1943, the Internal Revenue Service ruled that employee-based health coverage should be tax-free. At this point we were in the midst of the 1948 Declaration of Human Rights, but we were already heavy involved in the commodity-based insurance game.

→ Since then, access to healthcare in the United States has been handled through insurance, and because of this, most past reform efforts have been about insurance reform of some type, as seen on the following page:

1. Medicare/Medicaid 1965

↘

2. ERISA/COBRA 1974

↙

3. HIPAA 1996

↘

4. ACA 2010

⭐ **All four attempts have been noted to be movements towards increasing healthcare coverage and ending abuses of insurers.**

Be An Advocate

In Germany, their healthcare system is multi-payer because they use an employer-based system similar to ours. However, they are able to achieve Universal Health Coverage; three distinctions are upheld. Tight regulation gives the government much of the cost-control clout that the single-payer system provides. Health insurance plans have to cover everybody and cannot make a profit, and those who do not work and cannot afford to pay out-of-pocket receive public assistance to pay their premiums. Another big distinction Germany has is their cultural affirmation of safety-nets. They believe strongly, as a part of their German culture, to take care of the disadvantaged because they acknowledge and accept that anyone can fall into a disadvantaged state at any time. Professor Karl Lauterbach, a member of the German parliament, describes it as *"a system where the rich pay for the poor and where the ill are covered by the healthy. It's a social support system that is highly accepted by the population."*

They don't argue politically over whether or not to include a safety net because they accept its necessity and that healthcare is a right to all. It is no surprise that Germany has a higher life expectancy and lower infant mortality rate than we do.

I believe it is difficult for us to do this in the U.S. culturally because we aren't one culture here. We literally are the melting pot of the world, and as a result, have varying degrees of cultural beliefs on healthcare and access to it. Our melting pot is still stewing. We are not yet one cohesive stew in our beliefs. How else can we explain that we are the only country of every other developed country in the world that doesn't have some sort of universal health coverage for our citizens? Instead, our government allows healthcare companies to make a profit off of our health, which make some very rich, unlike any other comparable country in the world.

Single-payer, government-sponsored plans not only promise universal access but also, basic and essential benefits for every American. This allows us significant cost savings in exchange for more standardization, which includes reduced physician reimbursement and the repurposing of jobs in the health insurance sector. Some ways of approaching this can include government control, others can still include private insurers. The unfortunate circumstance in the great American healthcare debate is that our policymakers are fighting about how to take away healthcare from the poor because they can't pay for it.

Instead, the *overall* goal should be to *increase* coverage for everyone.

- -

We can debate about how to do it during elections and in congressional conversations. Until then, politicians who are representing the people of the United States take a unified and bi-partisan approach to Universal Health Coverage and debate regarding the funding mechanisms and how we should do it rather than fighting about whether or not we should.

This is one opportunity where we can unite and get something meaningful done. Our elected policymakers must decide how much they value investments in our personal and community health. Remember, we are not isolated beings; we live in a society with others.

Therefore, an investment in one is an investment in all.

The closest thing to single-payer already working and established in the U.S. is Medicare, which is where the concept of Medicare-for-all comes from. The infrastructure is already built, so it saves time and, subsequently, our taxpayer dollars. Medicare was established in 1965 under Title XVIII of the Social Security Act to provide health insurance to all people ages 65 and older, regardless of income or medical history.

This is in direct alignment with the goal of the United Nations Declaration of Human Rights of 1948. Since then, the United States has only acknowledged this human right for seniors, anyone over the age of 65, and no one else. The program has been expanded many times in the past to include people under 65 with end-stage renal disease (ESRD) and those with amyotrophic lateral sclerosis (ALS or Lou Gehrig's disease).

We seem capable of expanding coverage for those who are really sick but not for those who are poor. Medicare eligibility can be further expanded to help all people. Everyone who is working already pays for Medicare in their payroll taxes. This can be changed to be paid once a year during tax time. Options are available.

Be An Advocate

It is often argued that Medicare-for-all would make us bankrupt and broke. What people often miss is that although taxes will increase, our out-of-pocket monthly premiums will be eliminated. Forbes reports that "for the country as a whole this would largely be a financial wash." This is in addition to what was noted earlier; we are already paying way more than other countries are paying for universal coverage and wasting money away in inefficiencies. Some form of Medicare expansion will not bankrupt us. Yes, it will stop corporations from profiting off of us, which will make them upset, and as a result, they are the biggest opponents of Medicare expansions.

The trade-offs of Medicare-for-all will take time but can happen with better efficiencies and usage of taxpayer dollars. I'm already paying $700 a month for a health policy through my employer that gives it to Aetna, my health insurance plan, for me. I'd rather it be given to a federal system that will not profit off of me. Single-payer systems like Medicare-for-all will not be perfect but will solve some of our fiscal and ethical dilemmas because it would be controlled by a government entity with public oversight and not a giant corporation that does not have our best interests in mind.

Isn't that the *purpose* of electing our politicians and having a government—so they can <u>represent</u> our *best* interests?

At least that was the point of our founding Constitution.

- -

We could also keep private insurers and expand Medicare to all through the use of Medicare Advantage plans, which are already developed, effective, and working. These are private insurance plans offered to Medicare beneficiaries that include additional coverage not covered by traditional Medicare. Private insurance plans that offer Medicare Advantage must compete with one another for Medicare's business, which takes a market-oriented approach to competition and pricing.

Be An Advocate

The Affordable Care Act put some regulations in place that required private insurance companies offering these plans to follow in order to help contain costs and maintain solvency—all in the interest of its beneficiaries (all of us who pay into the system for many years).

A study published in Health Affairs found that Medicare Advantage plans, with the Federal regulation they have, cost less and deliver higher quality care than traditional Medicare.

We can work out a deal with private insurance companies that wins for all stakeholders. Additionally, we get more of a choice, the right to health, to be one of several hundred million potential voters to help shape its structure, and to become the true customer of American healthcare.

This last component is extremely important because anyone under the age of 65 that has private health insurance is not the true customer in American healthcare. Large and small group employers are. Insurance companies don't sell to us. Their plans are developed, designed, and marketed to the needs of employers, not consumers.

Medicare Advantage plans are the only health plans, other than the ones on the state marketplaces and sold through brokers, that are targeted and developed for the individual. In an era of disruption, innovation, and entrepreneurship, health plans that are focused on individuals will emerge and be designed to accommodate individual needs. What we demand and want in healthcare will naturally arise from consumer demand when the individual is the customer. As health plans get disrupted, so will our providers who will regain autonomy and provide services that are designed to work the best for us, not designed so that they are reimbursed the most by insurance.

Expanding Medicaid coverage works, too, but there are too many problems with the system because of its complexity between Federal, state, and managed care. If this complex system is simplified by getting rid of state regulation and moving toward standardized Federal regulation, then expanding Medicaid coverage through various programs, such as buy-ins, can work in the same fashion.

But why keep the young and the old citizens separate? Why have Medicaid for under 65 and Medicare for over 65?

Be An Advocate

It makes more sense to combine the two into one system for all of the complex reasons stated earlier, but also, it allows the older to spread their risk amongst everyone, including the much, much younger. In the same fashion as how large employer group plans are cheaper because they can spread the risk more, we can spread the risk amongst everyone in the country. Instead, we currently spread the risk amongst the poor (Medicaid) and the elderly (Medicare) in separate risk pools and wonder why we can't control costs.

Some states are considering implementing work requirements if they increase Medicaid coverage, but what doesn't make sense is that that is a form of paternalism. Telling people they need to work because it's right for them is unethical and immoral. Some people don't work because they must stay at home and care for a family member or their kids, so another parent can work. These are just more restrictions to not have to cover people, which is the opposite of what most state's public health goals are. Policymakers attempt to use state law to override Federal law not to increase coverage but, instead, add ways to reduce it.

Increasing **coverage will have impacts on our healthcare system, but the benefits** *highly* **outweigh the** *disadvantages*.

Be An Advocate

I want to briefly touch upon the understanding that single-payer or Medicare-for-all programs will force physicians and other providers to take the biggest hit initially. However, providers have directly influenced our current situation. How we reimburse them needs to evolve.

The fee-for-service reimbursement mechanism has pushed providers into a volume-based mindset, which is why they see us for the short periods of time that they do. The Physicians Foundation surveyed U.S. doctors and found that about 40% see 11 to 20 patients per day and 27% see 20 to 30 a day. A forum of nurses noted that they attend an average of 18 colonoscopies a day. We will no doubt have better health outcomes if our doctors spend more quality time with us and take interest in our health, instead of viewing us as quotas they need to meet.

Currently, the system is not tailored to the right incentives.

We often look to doctors as if they are gods without fault, but there is a reason why medical mistakes persist as the number three killer in the U.S.—third only to heart disease and cancer.

Providers need a serious reality check; perhaps taking smaller salaries, because what they provide is a public good and right to humans, should be considered. Absolutely, we should reform medical education to assist with the cost of tuition to help with this situation, but doctors have a duty to their fellow humans, and maybe we need more ethical doctors who follow the oaths they take in medical school.

Physicians that have high quality scores and do well with their patients, just like any other business, will succeed and do just fine. We want the low-performing doctors that have high complication rates to stop getting paid the same as doctors with high quality scores and, instead, go out of business. Providers have been insulated from this market-based competition, and maybe that's exactly what they need. Remember the old adage:

> *"What do you call the person that graduates the lowest in their class from Medical School? Doctor."*

We, as consumers, are the only ones who can provide the pressure needed to force this type of market-based change.

→ **Change** is what we need.

→ Let's start **asking** for it.

→ Be an **advocate** for a better healthcare system for everyone.

→ **Advocacy** is a powerful catalyst for the change we want to see.

→ Advocacy is any **action** that speaks in favor of, argues for a cause, or pleads on behalf of others.

→ It includes **educating** yourself, regulatory work, litigation, voting, and more.

→ Some representatives and politicians do **listen** to their constituents.

→ Reflect on and advocate for causes you support.

→ Make your **voice** heard in the voting booth and let Congress know what's important to you.

→ Every time you **speak** up for yourself or others, you are an advocate, and our healthcare system is in need of advocates.

→ You have the **power**. We can make **change**. Our time is **now**.

Afterword

Awareness

Dominates

Ignorance

In 2016, a good friend of mine asked me to give a presentation at her job for their weekly community learning and sharing program. Every Friday, the large corporate company held space for people to give talks about topics they are passionate about as learning opportunities for their employees. My friend, knowing that I was very enthusiastic about public health, asked me if I would. I jumped on the opportunity and looked at it as a public service to inform a small group of people about what was going on in our healthcare system. Everything was scheduled and ready to go. The day before, a notice went out to the employees at that organization's location, inviting them to my talk and providing a brief description of what the talk would be about. Several executives at the company caught wind of my talk's description and asked for my presentation ahead of time. After reviewing it, they canceled it, stating that the topic was too political. From that point on, I was determined to still get my presentation out, to provide opportunities for Americans to become informed about major healthcare issues that affect them directly, and to help spark a conversation amongst ourselves. This book is an output of that original presentation. From the very beginning, those supporting the status quo have been pushing back, attempting to keep the information in this book hidden, and making healthcare look like a taboo subject, never to be openly discussed. Our health is much more than just a political subject. It's our livelihood, our quality of life, and impacts everything from our personal bank accounts to our national economics.

Education is one of the most powerful things in life. It allows us to find meaning, gives us an understanding of the world around us, and offers us an opportunity to use the knowledge we gain wisely. Without education, that opportunity is stripped away from us. When we are informed and educated on something, we become equal. Barriers are removed, and common ground is laid for constructive conversation. Information makes us liberated and is the foundation of progress. What some are afraid of is that knowledge is power. If healthcare consumers become knowledgeable, they have power, and that power can impact our healthcare system. It is my hope that you will share this book with someone you love, and help them become an informed healthcare consumer in a battle against those who wish to keep this information undisclosed.

"The Mind

Once Enlightened

→ Thomas Paine

Can Never

Be Dark Again"

About The Series

Although the United States pays more for medical care than any other country, problems thrive in our healthcare system. Unsustainable costs, poor outcomes, high rates of medical errors, subpar patient satisfaction, and worsening health disparities all point to a need for change and reform efforts that must continue. Some progress has been made since the implementation of Medicare in the 40s to the Affordable Care Act of the present. However, much still needs to be done. Small incremental changes in healthcare policy won't suffice any longer. Paradigm shifting change is needed. This will not happen until pressure is put on those in the status quo by Americans becoming more informed and knowledgeable about our healthcare system.

Thought Collection Publishing's healthcare reform project aims to discuss the current state of our healthcare system in the fight to keep our healthcare system from collapsing and re-telling stories along the way. It has a goal that is two-fold. First, to educate the general population about our healthcare industry and turn consumers into educated people that ask questions and are informed about an industry we are born into, live with, and die in. Second, is to spark continued conversation among citizens and policymakers in an effort to discuss potential next steps in transforming healthcare. The overall message of our project is for better alignment around national solutions for the health of our communities. We have to move from thinking individually and in small groups to thinking universally. If we can align our efforts around the common goal of creating healthy communities, we can stop our system from collapsing.

Thought Collection Publishing has dedicated its healthcare reform project to advocate for awareness and a person's right to know. It is time for America's healthcare woes to be diagnosed, healed, and for the system to become accountable and change for the better. This book series will spread the truth about healthcare in the U.S. and defend a position for a better system for us all. 90% of the general public is unaware of their rights as patients and healthcare consumers, as well as of the inner-workings of the system they use for their entire life. This book series looks to bridge this gap by removing the conditioned ignorance that exists.

Educated health consumers = pressure = competition & policy change = affordability & equity.

www.ToErrIsHealthcare.com
www.InformedHealthConsumer.com
Join the mailing list at www.eepurl.com/Tk0XD

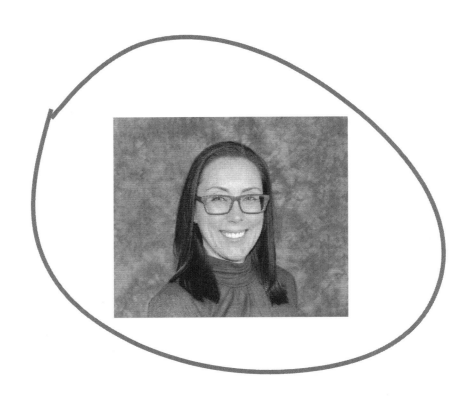

Meet The Author!

Kat is an award-winning writer, educator, reformer, health advocate, and believer of healthcare as a human right. She holds an MBA and is an inductee of Sigma Beta Delta, the National Honor Society in Business, Management, and Administration. As an Adjunct Professor, she became very passionate about educating the community about health policy and the current social issues that plague the industry. Her passion for public health has given her appointment by a former Illinois Governor on the State Health Improvement Planning and Healthy Illinois 2021 Planning councils where she hopes to positively influence health policy. She believes that most of us aren't comfortable watching people suffer when help is available, and when we assist each other in surviving, everyone benefits. She advocates for awareness, transparency, and a person's right to know.

Connect With Her!

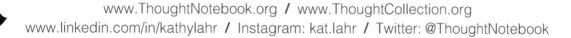

www.ThoughtNotebook.org / www.ThoughtCollection.org
www.linkedin.com/in/kathylahr / Instagram: kat.lahr / Twitter: @ThoughtNotebook

& Continue The Mission!

Join Kat's Facebook group and be a part of a community of Americans who want to be informed health consumers. Be a resource to each other as we all embark together on the learning curve of becoming more educated and aware of the happenings in our health system. Become active in important healthcare discussions and begin to gain back your influence and power over the system we are born into, live, and die in.

www.facebook.com/groups/informedhealthconsumer

Kat has developed discussion notes for book clubs and reading groups to continue the conversation locally in their small groups. Download them at:

www.toerrishealthcare.com/for-book-clubs

Acknowledgements

This book would have never been possible without the help of many people. I'd like to thank them for their support and love of this project.

To my husband, Tom, and daughter, Dez, for their continued support and sacrifice to help make my dream of publishing this book come true and for their unwavering acknowledgement of the fire I have inside that fuels my passion for equity in healthcare and public health.

To my editing intern, Miranda Malinowski, for helping me blaze my words so that their complexity can make the right impact and be digestible to those who read it. To my design intern, Davis Smith, for bringing my vision to fiery life and infusing it with an innovative approach to visual learning. Both of your sacrifices of time and energy have meant the world to me and will be impactful to our healthcare system.

To my healthcare management students for showing me the tremendous opportunity that awaits for educating Americans in healthcare system knowledge. Your eagerness to devour more, go deeper, and take action inspired me to share with others outside of the four walls of the classroom.

To all of the researchers who I have used as sources to obtain knowledge, thank you for your time and energy to bring luminosity to areas that need to be understood better. You have charged up and awakened areas within me that sat dormant. You have sparked my curiosity which has been summoned into advocacy. Your research has, and will continue to, start thought-provoking conversation.

To Erin Brockovich, Angela Davis, Sophocles, and Audre Lorde, for bringing me continued inspiration and fuel to keep the fires of change lit strongly within me. Your words have illuminated my thoughts and made me realize that being radical is what's required.

To you, reader, for taking the time to read and learn more about something so intimate to us all. Your time spent learning will help us make an unstoppable inferno of awareness and change.

Sources Part 1

→ Agency for Healthcare Research and Quality. Hospital Guide to Reducing Medicaid Readmissions, U.S. Department of Health and Human Services, August 2014, https://www.ahrq.gov/sites/default/files/publications/files/medreadmissions.pdf.

→ Bradley, S and McDermott, D. How Do Mortality Rates in the U.S. Compare To Other Countries, Kaiser Family Foundation, February 2019, https://www.healthsystemtracker.org/chart-collection/mortality-rates-u-s-compare-countries/#item-start.

→ Centers for Disease Control and Prevention. Leading Causes of Death, National Center for Health Statistics, https://www.cdc.gov/nchs/fastats/leading-causes-of-death.htm.

→ Conway, P. 49 States Plus DC Reduce Avoidable Hospital Readmissions, Centers For Medicare and Medicaid, September 2013, https://blog.cms.gov/2016/09/13/new-data-49-states-plus-dc-reduce-avoidable-hospital-readmissions/.

→ Commonwealth Fund. Spending on Health Insurance Administration Per Capita. Multinational Comparisons of Health Systems Data, November 2014, https://www.commonwealthfund.org/chart/2014/spending-health-insurance-administration-capita.

→ Coyne College. The Cost of Childbirth Across The Globe, https://www.slideshare.net/brianahier/international-federation-of-health-plans-price-report.

→ Dana O., et al. Paying for Prescription Drugs Around the World: Why Is The U.S. An Outlier?, The Commonwealth Fund, October 2017, https://www.commonwealthfund.org/publications/issue-briefs/2017/oct/paying-prescription-drugs-around-world-why-us-outlier.

→ Department of Health and Human Services. America's Health Literacy: Why We Need Accessible Health Information, Office of Disease Prevention and Health Promotion, Health Communication Activities, 2008, https://health.gov/communication/literacy/issuebrief/#survey.

→ Dobson, A., et al. Use of Home Health Care and Other Care Services Among Medicare Beneficiaries, Alliance for Home Health Quality and Innovation, July 2012, http://www.ahhqi.org/images/pdf/cacep-wp4-baselines.pdf.

→ Fontana, E. and Hawes, K. Map: See The 2,599 Hospitals That Will Face Readmissions Penalties This Year, Advisory Board, September 2018, https://www.advisory.com/daily-briefing/2018/09/27/readmissions.

→ Gonzales, S., et al. How Does U.S. Life Expectancy Compare To Other Countries? Peterson-Kaiser Health System Tracker, Chart Collections Health & Wellbeing, April 2019, https://www.healthsystemtracker.org/chart-collection/u-s-life-expectancy-compare-countries/#item-start.

→ Himmelstein, D, et al. A Comparison of Hospital Administrative Costs In Eight Nations: US Costs Exceed All Others By Far, Health Affairs 33, No. 9., September 2014, https://www.healthaffairs.org/doi/full/10.1377/hlthaff.2013.1327.

→ International Federation of Health Plans. 2012 Comparative Price Report: Variation in Medical and Hospital Prices by Country, Harvard, 2012, http://hushp.harvard.edu/sites/default/files/downloadable_files/IFHP%202012%20Comparative%20Price%20Report.pdf.

→ James, J. A New, Evidence-based Estimate of Patient Harms Associated with Hospital Care, Journal of Patient Safety: September 2013, https://journals.lww.com/journalpatientsafety/Fulltext/2013/09000/A_New,_Evidence_based_Estimate_of_Patient_Harms.2.aspx.

→ Jordan, R. Medicare Eases Readmission Penalties Against Safety-Net Hospitals, Kaiser Health News, September 2018, https://khn.org/news/medicare-eases-readmissions-penalties-against-safety-net-hospitals/.

→ Kamal, R. and Cox, C. How Do Healthcare Prices and Use in the U.S. Compare to Other Countries, Kaiser Family Foundation, May 2018, https://www.healthsystemtracker.org/chart-collection/how-do-healthcare-prices-and-use-in-the-u-s-compare-to-other-countries/#item-the-average-price-of-an-mri-in-the-u-s-is-significantly-higher-than-in-comparable-countries_2018.

→ MedPAC. The Hospital Readmissions Reduction Program Has Succeeded for Beneficiaries and the Medicare Program, Medicare Payment Advisory Commission, June 2018, http://www.medpac.gov/-blog-/the-hospital-readmissions-reduction-program-(hrrp)-has-succeeded-for-beneficiaries-and-the-medicare-program/2018/06/15/the-hospital-readmissions-reduction-program-has-succeeded-for-beneficiaries-and-the-medicare-program.

→ Mercola, J. 10 Shocking Medical Mistakes, June 2012, https://articles.mercola.com/sites/articles/archive/2012/06/27/top-10-medical-mistakes.aspx.

→ Michael, D. Study Suggests Medical Errors Now Third Leading Cause of Death in the U.S., May 2016, https://www.hopkinsmedicine.org/news/media/releases/study_suggests_medical_errors_now_third_leading_cause_of_death_in_the_us.

→ National Academies of Sciences, Engineering, and Medicine. Improving Diagnosis in Health Care, September, 2015, http://www.nationalacademies.org/hmd/reports/2015/improving-diagnosis-in-healthcare.

→ Noss, A. Household Income: 2012, United States Census Report, September 2013, https://www.census.gov/library/publications/2013/acs/acsbr12-02.html.

→ OECD. OECD Factbook 2015-2016: Economic, Environmental and Social Statistics, OECD Publishing, 2016, https://doi.org/10.1787/factbook-2015-86-en.

→ OECD. Health at a Glance 2017, OECD Publishing, November 2017, https://doi.org/10.1787/health_glance-2017-en.

→ OECD. Health Statistics 2019, OECD Publishing, July 2019, https://www.oecd.org/els/health-systems/health-data.htm.

→ OECD 2017. "Infant health" in Health at a Glance 2017: OECD Indicators, OECD Publishing, https://doi.org/10.1787/health_glance-2017-11-en.

→ OECD. Life expectancy at birth and health spending per capita, 2015, Health Status, OECD Publishing, 2017, https://doi.org/10.1787/health_glance-2017-graph8-en.

→ OECD. Obesity Update 2017, OECD Publishing, 2017, https://www.oecd.org/health/obesity-update.htm.

→ OECD. Pharmaceutical Spending Indicator, Health Expenditure And Financing Database, July 2019, https://data.oecd.org/healthres/pharmaceutical-spending.htm.

→ Papanicolas, L. R. Woskie, L., Jha, A. Health Care Spending in the United States and Other High-Income Countries, Journal of the American Medical Association, March 2018, https://www.commonwealthfund.org/publications/journal-article/2018/mar/health-care-spending-united-states-and-other-high-income.

→ Save the Children Foundation. State of the World's Mothers: Surviving the First Day, Bill and Melinda Gates Foundation, May 2013, https://www.savethechildren.org/content/dam/usa/reports/advocacy/sowm/sowm-2013.pdf.

→ Save the Children Foundation. State of the World's Mothers: The Urban Disadvantage, Bill and Melinda Gates Foundation, May 2015, https://www.savethechildren.org/content/dam/usa/reports/advocacy/sowm/sowm-2015.pdf.

→ Sawyer, B. The average price of Copaxone in the U.S. is almost 3 times the average price in Switzerland, Peterson-Kaiser Health System Tracker, May 2017, https://www.healthsystemtracker.org/chart/average-price-copaxone-u-s-almost-3-times-average-price-switzerland/#item-start.

→ Schneider, E., et al. Mirror, Mirror 2017: International Comparison Reflects Flaws and Opportunities for Better U.S. Health Care, Commonwealth Fund, July 2017, https://interactives.commonwealthfund.org/2017/july/mirror-mirror/assets/Schneider_mirror_mirror_2017.pdf.

→ Squires, D. and Anderson, C. U.S. Health Care from a Global Perspective: Spending, Use of Services, Prices, and Health in 13 Countries, The Commonwealth Fund, October 2015, https://www.commonwealthfund.org/publications/issue-briefs/2015/oct/us-health-care-global-perspective?redirect_source=/publications/issue-briefs/2015/oct/us-health-care-from-a-global-perspective.

→ The State Of Obesity. National Obesity Rates & Trends, Robert Wood Johnson Foundation, 2019, https://www.stateofobesity.org/obesity-rates-trends-overview/.

→ Thomas, T., et al. Variation in Surgical-Readmission Rates and Quality of Hospital Care, N Engl J Med, September 2013, https://www.nejm.org/doi/full/10.1056/NEJMsa1303118.

Sources Part 1 (cont.)

→ United Nations. Universal Declaration of Human Rights, https://www.un.org/en/universal-declaration-human-rights.

→ United States Senate. More than 1,000 preventable deaths a day is too many: the need to improve patient safety, Subcommittee on Primary Health and Aging of the Committee on Health, Education, Labor, and Pensions, July 2014, https://www.govinfo.gov/content/pkg/CHRG-113shrg88894/pdf/CHRG-113shrg88894.pdf.

→ Wei, S., Olga, P., Allen, M. Surgeon Scorecard, ProPublica, July 2015, https://projects.propublica.org/surgeons.

→ Woolhandler, S. et al. Costs of Health Care Administration in the United States and Canada, N Engl J Med, August 2003, https://www.nejm.org/doi/full/10.1056/nejmsa022033.

→ Zuckerman, R., et al. Readmissions, Observation, and the Hospital Readmissions Reduction Program, N Engl J Med, April 2016, https://www.nejm.org/doi/pdf/10.1056/NEJMsa1513024.

Sources Part 2

→ Associated Press. Health Care CEOs Again Lead The Way In Pay, May 2019, https://www.apnews.com/c3febcd7d7bc4d909db2db-d50604abd0.

→ Barnsteiner, J. Patient Safety and Quality: An Evidence-Based Handbook for Nurses, Agency for Healthcare Research and Quality, April 2008, https://www.ncbi.nlm.nih.gov/books/NBK2648.

→ Curtin, L. Ethics case study: Just Watch Them Die, American Nurse Today Vol. 10 No. 4, April 2015, https://www.americannursetoday.com/ethics-case-study-just-watch-die/.

→ Federalpay.org. Federal Employee Lookup: Seema Verma, 2017, https://www.federalpay.org/employees/centers-for-medicare-and-medicaid-services/verma-seema.

→ Duffin, E. Average Annual CEO Compensation Worldwide In 2017, Statista, April 2019, https://www.statista.com/statistics/424154/average-annual-ceo-compensation-worldwide.

→ Institute For Policy Studies. CEO-Worker Pay Resource Guide, 2019, https://inequality.org/action/corporate-pay-equity.

→ Kurutkan, M., et al. An Implementation On The Social Cost Of Hospital Acquired Infections, International Journal of Clinical and Experimental Medicine, March 2015, https://www.ncbi.nlm.nih.gov/pmc/articles/PMC4443201.

→ Herman, B. The Sky-High Pay of Health Care CEOs, Axios, December 2017, https://www.axios.com/the-sky-high-pay-of-health-care-ceos-1513303956-d5b874a8-b4a0-4e74-9087-353a2ef1ba83.html.

→ Healthcare Finance. Changing Of CEO Guard at Blues Giant HCSC, July 2015, https://www.healthcarefinancenews.com/news/changing-ceo-guard-blues-giant-hcsc.

→ Herman, Bob. Executive Pay At Health Care Service Corp Rises Despite ACA Troubles, Modern Healthcare, September 2016, https://www.modernhealthcare.com/article/20160926/NEWS/160929921/executive-pay-at-health-care-service-corp-rises-despite-aca-troubles.

→ Joynt, K., et al. Compensation Of Chief Executive Officers At Nonprofit US Hospitals, JAMA Internal Medicine, January 2014, https://jamanetwork.com/journals/jamainternalmedicine/fullarticle/1748832.

→ Kacik, A. Community Health Systems Unit Settles False-Billing Case for $262M, Modern Healthcare, September 2018, https://www.modernhealthcare.com/article/20180925/NEWS/180929922/community-health-systems-unit-settles-false-billing-case-for-262m.

→ Kaiser Health News. Hospital CEO Pay And Incentives, June 2013, https://khn.org/news/hospital-ceo-compensation-chart.

→ Rege, A. Universal Health Services CEO Make 541x More Than Average Employee, Becker's Hospital Review, April 2018, https://www.beckershospitalreview.com/compensation-issues/universal-health-services-ceo-made-541x-more-than-average-employee.html.

→ West Health. The U.S. Healthcare Cost Crisis, Gallup, 2019, https://news.gallup.com/poll/248081/westhealth-gallup-us-healthcare-cost-crisis.aspx.

→ Wood, M., et al. Executive Excess 2014: The Obamacare Prescription For Bloated CEO Pay, Institute For Policy Studies, August 2014, https://ips-dc.org/obamacare-prescription.

Sources Part 3

→ AllNurses. How Many Colonoscopies Per Day?, Gastroenterology Forum, December 2009, https://allnurses.com/many-colonoscopies-per-day-t311379.

→ American Hospital Association. Uncompensated Hospital Care Cost Fact Sheet, January 2019, https://www.aha.org/fact-sheet/2019-01-02-uncompensated-hospital-care-cost-fact-sheet-january-2019.

→ American Medical Association. Ethics: Informed Consent, AMA Principles of Medical Ethics: I, II, V, VIII, 2019, https://www.ama-assn.org/delivering-care/ethics/informed-consent.

→ Association of American Medical Colleges. New Findings Confirm Predictions on Physician Shortage, AAMC News, April 2019, https://news.aamc.org/press-releases/article/2019-workforce-projections-update.

→ Barbey, C., et al. Physician Workforce Trends and Their Implications for Spending Growth, Health Affairs, July 2018, https://www.healthaffairs.org/do/10.1377/hblog20170728.061252/full.

→ Berchick, E., et al. Health Insurance Coverage in the United States: 2017, U.S. Dept of Commerce, September 2018, https://www.census.gov/content/dam/Census/library/publications/2018/demo/p60-264.pdf.

→ Campos, M. Leaky Gut: What Is It, And What Does It Mean For You?, Harvard Health Publishing, September 2017, https://www.health.harvard.edu/blog/leaky-gut-what-is-it-and-what-does-it-mean-for-you-2017092212451.

→ Centers for Disease Control and Prevention. State Physical Activity and Nutrition Program Recipients, May 2019, https://www.cdc.gov/nccdphp/dnpao/state-local-programs/span-1807/span-1807-recipients.html.

→ Centers for Medicare and Medicaid Services. CAHPS Overview, HCAHPS: Patients' Perspectives of Care Survey, March 2017, https://www.cms.gov/Medicare/Quality-Initiatives-Patient-Assessment-Instruments/HospitalQualityInits/HospitalHCAHPS.html.

→ Centers for Medicare and Medicaid Services. Historical National Health Expenditure Data, December 2018, https://www.cms.gov/Research-Statistics-Data-and-Systems/Statistics-Trends-and-Reports/NationalHealthExpendData/NationalHealthAccountsHistorical.html.

→ Centers for Medicare and Medicaid Services. National Health Expenditure Data: Historical, November 2018, https://www.cms.gov/research-statistics-data-and-systems/statistics-trends-and-reports/nationalhealthexpenddata/nationalhealthaccountshistorical.html.

→ Centers for Medicare and Medicaid Services. The Affordable Care Act: Increasing Transparency, Protecting Consumers, The Center for Consumer Information & Insurance Oversight, 2019, https://www.cms.gov/CCIIO/Resources/Fact-Sheets-and-FAQs/increasing-transparency02162012a.html.

→ Chaussee, J. Ban on Inmate Sterilizations Moves Forward In California Legislature, Reuters, June 2014, https://www.reuters.com/article/us-usa-california-prisons/ban-on-inmate-sterilizations-moves-forward-in-california-legislature-idUSKBN0F008A20140625.

Sources Part 3 (cont.)

→ Cordina, J., et al. Healthcare Consumerism 2018: An Update on the Journey, McKinsey, July 2018, https://www.mckinsey.com/industries/healthcare-systems-and-services/our-insights/healthcare-consumerism-2018.

→ Coughlin, T., et al. Uncompensated Care for the Uninsured in 2013: A Detailed Examination, Kaiser Family Foundation, https://www.kff.org/uninsured/report/uncompensated-care-for-the-uninsured-in-2013-a-detailed-examination/view/print.

→ Dartmouth Atlas of Health Care Working Group. The Care Of Patients With Severe Chronic Illness: An Online Report On The Medicare Program, The Dartmouth Atlas Project, 2006, http://archive.dartmouthatlas.org/downloads/atlases/2006_Chronic_Care_Atlas.pdf.

→ Dizioli, Allan and Pinheiro, Roberto B. Health Insurance as a Productive Factor, University of Pennsylvania and University of Colorado, 2012, https://mpra.ub.uni-muenchen.de/39743.

→ Fields, H. The Gut: Where Bacteria and Immune System Meet, John Hopkins Medicine, November 2015, https://www.hopkinsmedicine.org/research/advancements-in-research/fundamentals/in-depth/the-gut-where-bacteria-and-immune-system-meet.

→ Goodman, J. What You Need To Know About Medicare For All, Forbes, September 2018, https://www.forbes.com/sites/johngoodman/2018/09/07/what-you-need-to-know-about-medicare-for-all-part-i/#4d62755373d3.

→ Huckfelt, P. Less Intense Postacute Care, Better Outcomes For Enrollees In Medicare Advantage Than Those In Fee-For-Service, Health Affairs, January 2017, https://www.healthaffairs.org/doi/pdf/10.1377/hlthaff.2016.1027.

→ Jiwani, A., et al. Billing and Insurance-Related Administrative Costs in United States' Health Care: Synthesis of Micro-Costing Evidence, BMC Health Services Research, 2014, https://bmchealthservres.biomedcentral.com/track/pdf/10.1186/s12913-014-0556-7.

→ Insurance Information Institute. Facts + Statistics: Industry Overview, 2019, https://www.iii.org/fact-statistic/facts-statistics-industry-overview.

→ IPSOS. Ipsos/NPR Data: Healthcare Knowledge and Perception, NPR, January 2017, https://www.ipsos.com/en-us/news-polls/ipsos-npr-data-healthcare-knowledge-and-perception.

→ John Hopkins Medicine. Study Suggests Medical Errors Now Third Leading Cause of Death in the U.S., May 2016, https://www.hopkinsmedicine.org/news/media/releases/study_suggests_medical_errors_now_third_leading_cause_of_death_in_the_us.

→ Kaiser Family Foundation. Key Facts about the Uninsured Population, December 2018, https://www.kff.org/uninsured/fact-sheet/key-facts-about-the-uninsured-population.

→ Kaiser Family Foundation. Kaiser Health Tracking Poll, March 2013, https://www.kff.org/health-reform/poll-finding/march-2013-tracking-poll.

→ Kane, L. Medscape Physician Compensation Report 2019, Medscape, https://www.medscape.com/slideshow/2019-compensation-overview-6011286#3.

→ Kochanek, K. Mortality in the United States, CDC's National Center for Health Statistics, December 2017, https://www.cdc.gov/nchs/data/databriefs/db293.pdf.

→ Lassler, K., et al. Access to Care, Health Status, and Health Disparities in the United States and Canada: Results of a Cross-National Population-Based Survey, American Journal of Public Health, 2006, https://www.ncbi.nlm.nih.gov/pmc/articles/PMC1483879.

→ Masters R., et all. Return on Investment of Public Health Interventions: A Systematic Review, Journal of Epidemiology and Community Health, 2017, http://jech.bmj.com/content/jech/early/2017/03/07/jech-2016-208141.full.

→ McKillop, M., et al. The Impact Of Chronic Underfunding On America's Public Health System: Trends, Risks, and Recommendations, Trust For America's Health, 2019, https://www.tfah.org/wp-content/uploads/2019/04/TFAH-2019-PublicHealthFunding-06.pdf.

→ Mitchell A and Heisler E. Bipartisan Budget Act of 2018: CHIP, Public Health, Home Visiting, and Medicaid Provisions in Division E, Congressional Research Service, March 2018, https://fas.org/sgp/crs/misc/R45136.pdf.

→ Mokdad, A., et al. Actual Causes of Death in the United States, JAMA, March 2000, https://jamanetwork.com/journals/jama/article-abstract/198357.

→ National Academies of Sciences, Engineering and Medicine. Engineers and Health Professionals Should Work Together To Address Quality and Cost of Health Care, News From The National Academies, July 2005, http://www8.nationalacademies.org/onpinews/newsitem.aspx?RecordID=11378.

→ National Health Care Anti-Fraud Association. The Challenge of Health Care Fraud, 2018, https://www.nhcaa.org/resources/health-care-anti-fraud-resources/the-challenge-of-health-care-fraud.aspx.

→ National Prevention Council. National Prevention Strategy, U.S. Department of Health and Human Services, Office of the Surgeon General, 2011, https://www.hhs.gov/sites/default/files/disease-prevention-wellness-report.pdf.

→ Office of the National Coordinator for Health Information Technology. Your Health Information, Your Rights, October 2015, https://www.healthit.gov/sites/default/files/YourHealthInformationYourRights_Infographic-Web.pdf.

→ Organization for Economic Cooperation and Development. OECD Health Statistics: Social Protection, OECD Library, July 2019, https://www.oecd-ilibrary.org/social-issues-migration-health/data/oecd-health-statistics/oecd-health-data-social-protection_data-00544-en?parentId=http%3A%2F%2Finstance.metastore.ingenta.com%2Fcontent%2Fcollection%2Fhealth-data-en.

→ Palfreman, J. Sick Around The World, PBS Frontline, April 2008, https://www.pbs.org/wgbh/frontline/film/sickaroundtheworld.

→ Patel, W., et al. Trends in Consumer Access and Use of Electronic Health Information, The Office of the National Coordinator for Health Information Technology, October 2015, https://dashboard.healthit.gov/evaluations/data-briefs/trends-consumer-access-use-electronic-health-information.php.

→ Peterson-Kaiser. Health System Tracker: Health Determinants, 2019, https://www.healthsystemtracker.org/indicator/health-well-being/poverty-status.

→ Physicians for a National Health Program. Health Care Systems - Four Basic Models, 2010, http://www.pnhp.org/single_payer_resources/health_care_systems_four_basic_models.php.

→ Physicians Foundation. A Survey of America's Physicians: Practice Patterns and Perspectives, September 2012, https://physiciansfoundation.org/focus-areas/a-survey-of-americas-physicians-practice-patterns-and-perspectives.

→ Starfield, B., et al. Contribution of Primary Care to Health Systems and Health, The Milbank Quarterly, September 2005, https://www.ncbi.nlm.nih.gov/pmc/articles/PMC2690145.

→ State Of Illinois. State Budget Fiscal Year 2020, February 2019, https://www2.illinois.gov/sites/budget/Documents/Budget%20Book/FY2020-Budget-Book/Fiscal-Year-2020-Operating-Budget-Book.pdf.

→ Stuckler, D., et al. The political economy of universal health coverage. World Health Organization, November 2010, https://researchonline.lshtm.ac.uk/id/eprint/2157.

→ U.S. Census Bureau. Percentage of Children Under Age 19 and Adults Aged 19 to 64 Without Health Insurance Coverage by Selected Characteristics, Current Population Survey, 2017, https://www.census.gov/content/dam/Census/library/visualizations/2017/demo/p60-260/figure6.pdf.

→ U.S. Census Bureau. Uninsured Rate by State, Current Population Survey, 2017, https://www.census.gov/content/dam/Census/library/visualizations/2018/demo/p60-264/figure7.pdf.

→ U.S. Census Bureau. Uninsured Rate by Poverty Status and Medicaid Expansion of State for Adults Aged 19 to 64, Current Population Survey, 2017, https://www.census.gov/content/dam/Census/library/visualizations/2018/demo/p60-264/figure5.pdf.

Sources Part 3 (cont.)

→ U.S. Census Bureau. Uninsured Rate by Single Year of Age, Current Population Survey, 2017, https://www.census.gov/content/dam/Census/library/visualizations/2018/demo/p60-264/figure4.pdf.

→ United States Senate. Concurrent and Overlapping Surgeries: Additional Measures Warranted, A Senate Finance Committee Staff Report, December 2016, https://www.finance.senate.gov/imo/media/doc/Concurrent%20Surgeries%20Report%20Final.pdf.

→ West Health Institute. Americans' Views Of Healthcare Costs, Coverage, and Policy, University of Chicago, 2018, https://www.westhealth.org/wp-content/uploads/2018/03/WHI-Healthcare-Costs-Coverage-and-Policy-Issue-Brief.pdf

→ Wilper, A., et al. Health Insurance and Mortality in US Adults, American Journal of Public Health, December 2009, https://www.ncbi.nlm.nih.gov/pmc/articles/PMC2775760.

→ World Health Organization. Sustainable Development Goals: Universal Health Coverage, World Health Statistics, 2018, https://www.who.int/en/news-room/fact-sheets/detail/universal-health-coverage-(uhc).

→ Wu, H and Wu, E. The Role Of Gut Microbiota in Immune Homeostasis and Autoimmunity, Gut Microbes, January 2012, https://www.ncbi.nlm.nih.gov/pmc/articles/PMC3337124.

→ YMCA of Metropolitan Washington. YMCA's Diabetes Prevention Program, https://www.ymcadc.org/ymcas-diabetes-prevention-program/.

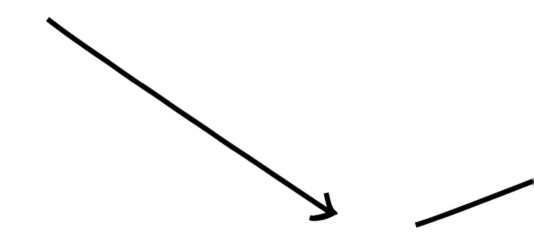

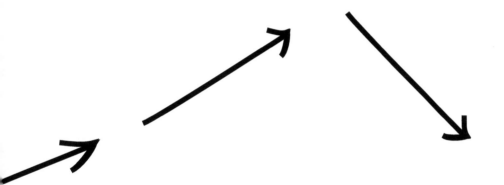

Don't Take My Research For Granted!
Do Your Own Too!

Made in the USA
Columbia, SC
30 January 2020

87311328R00130